OSCE & LMCC–II

Review Notes

Zu-hua Gao, MD, PhD, FRCPC

Editor

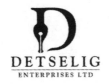

DETSELIG
ENTERPRISES LTD

Calgary, Alberta

OSCE & LMCC–II

© 2005 Zu-hua Gao

Library and Archives Canada Cataloguing in Publication

  OSCE & LMCC II : review notes / Zu-Hua Gao, editor.
ISBN 1-55059-301-3
  1. Clinical medicine – Examinations – Study guides.
2. Physicians – Licenses – Canada – Examinations – Study guides.
I. Gao, Zu-hua

R735.083 2005   616'.0076   C2005-904586-8

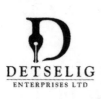

Detselig Enterprises Ltd.
210, 1220 Kensington Road NW
Calgary, Alberta T2N 3P5

Phone: (403) 283-0900
Fax: (403) 283-6947
Email: temeron@telusplanet.net
www.temerondetselig.com

We acknowledge the support of the Government of Canada through the Book Publishing Industry Development Program (BPIDP) for our publishing program.
We also acknowledge the support of the Alberta Foundation for the Arts for our publishing program.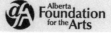

Cover design by Alvin Choong

ISBN 1-55059-301-3   SAN 113-0234   Printed in Canada

Preface

This *OSCE & LMCC–II: Review Notes* originated from collections of study notes that passed on from several resident training programs in Canada. It provides an unofficial guide for the preparation of LMCC Part II examination. It is also useful for the preparation of Clinical Skills Assessment examination for US residents.

This book presents approximately 200 most commonly encountered clinical scenarios. It not only helps you in the preparation of examination, but also helps you in your daily clinical practice. A word of advice is to practice these skills every time you see a patient in your clinical rotation. This study notes collection is by no means a complete official answer to any of these questions. However, it can be used as a framework where new information can be added. This book complements many texts that contain more in depth information about these clinical entities.

The author gratefully acknowledges the contribution of Dr. Chad Ball, Dr. Marjan Afrouzian, Dr. Javad Ahmadi, Dr. Peyman Saleheh Shoshtari, Michelle Chow and Yuan Gao. Without their help, this book would not have been possible.

Zu-hua Gao, MD, PhD, FRCPC

Contents

Steps for a Successful Examination

- **Study for the exam:**
1. To group with 3 or 4 candidates to practice the possible scenarios has proven to be very helpful. Keep tracking your time on each station during the practice.
2. Remember to verbalize every step you are doing in the physical exam, "speaking while doing."
3. View videotapes and DVD's in the library and try to mimic the clinical encounter of those physicians. I found some movies helpful as well, such as *Chicago Hope.*

- **Tips for the exam:**
1. Read the questions carefully. Be clear about the objectives of the station, such as *take a history, or provide consult,* etc.
2. Shake hands with your patient while introducing yourself.
3. Set the scene by telling the patient what you are going to do, or what topics you are going to discuss, etc.
4. Be empathic while addressing patients' symptoms. Address (verbally) potential discomfort before starting the physical examination.
5. Be focused and systematic to proceed with your questions or examinations.
6. Speak slowly, clearly, gentle but loud enough so that both patients and the examiner can hear you.
7. Mind your body language: don't fold your arms across the chest, or put a hand to the back of your neck. Try to make the patient comfortable by touching their arm or let an agitated patient sit down.
8. If you happened to forget what to ask next, do a few open questions such as: "Tell me more about . . .?" "Is there anything else bothering you?"
9. If you complete your questions or examinations early, try to fill the time by summarizing the information by saying "so you have told me . . . ," or by exploring other problems by saying "is everything else OK?"

10. Use "Do you have any other concerns or questions?" to indicate the end of the conversation. Address future contacts or communications with the patient by saying "I'd like to see you again in the few days to make sure the treatment is working well, etc."

11. Thank the patient (and the examiner) before leaving the room.

1
Family Medicine

1. Sexual Assault
Case 1.
Sexual assault victim. Take a history and manage.

Key:
Be sympathetic, respective. Presence of a nurse when examining a female patient.

History:
- *Who and how many?*
- *When?*
- *Where did penetration occur?*
- *What happened? Any weapons and physical assault?*
- *Any post assault activities? urination, defecation, change clothes, shower, douches, etc.*
- *When did the last voluntary intercourse occur?*
- *Gynecology history: G&P, LMP, contraception, AMPLE*
- *Address HIV, Hepatitis B, tetanus, pregnancy and physical trauma, vaccination and prevention.*

Management:
ABC first
- Ensure patient is not left alone and that ongoing emotional support is provided
- Set aside adequate time for exam (usually 1.5 hrs)
- <u>Obtain</u> <u>consent</u> <u>for:</u> medical exam and treatment, evidence collection; disclosure to police – notify police as soon as consent obtained
- Use sexual assault kit to ensure uniformity and completeness
- Chain of evidence: label samples immediately, pass directly to police.
- Offer community crisis resources e.g. shelter, hotline psychology referral
- Involve social workers

2. Violence Against Women

Case 1.
36 YOF, physically assaulted by her husband. Assess and manage.

Case 2.
Man presented to your office; he has hit his wife. Assess risk factors for physical abuse.

Key:
Recognition, evaluation, documentation and referral.

History:
- *Is this the first time you have hit your wife?*
- *What is the cause of this?*
- *Have you been abused or witnessed abuse when you were young?*
- *What is your social/economic status, ethnic background?*
- *Are you under any stress?*
- *Do you drink alcohol, how much? how frequently? Do you use drugs?*
- *How do you solve differences with your wife? with other people?*
- *How do you express or control anger?*
- *Is there lack of trust between you and your wife?*

Risk factors:
- Socioeconomic, educational and cultural background
- 80% male batterers were abused as children and had witnessed wife abuse in their family
- 67% battered women witnessed their mothers being abused
- ETOH may contribute to the violence as a facilitator but not the cause
- Assaultive men are often not violent outside home
- Rigid definitions of male/female roles are common
- Uses violence as a problem-solving technique
- Tendency towards excessive jealousy, lack of trust of partner or others

- Inability to express feelings except through anger, inability to control anger

Management:

Recognition

Physical:

1. Serious bleeding injury in trunk, bruises, welts, burns, dislocated or broken bones, torn ligaments, perforated ear drums, dental injuries
2. Frequent visits with non-specific complaints.

Psychological: anxiety attacks, crying spells, depression, suicidal thoughts, drug/alcohol abuse

Evaluation

- Interview women alone, use nonjudgmental direct questions
- Reinforce assault is crime, don't blame the women
- Ask about safety of children and women, has any child seen this violence

Documentation

- Physical trauma and psychological symptoms, quote patient directly
- Pictures are helpful

Referral

Social work:

- Ensure the patient has a safe environment to go to after disclosure
- Create an escape plan if the patient needs to leave abusive spouse

3. Skin Rashes/Blisters

Case 1.

21 YOF presented with skin rashes and blisters. Obtain a focused history and perform a physical exam in 10 minutes.

History:

- *Age, race, occupation, hobbies*
- *Is the onset sudden or gradual?*
- *Is the skin itchy or painful?*
- *Is there any discharge (blood or pus)?*
- *Where?*
- *Have you recently taken any antibiotics or other drug or topical meds?*
- *Were there any proceeding systemic symptoms? Fever, sore throat, anorexia, and/or vaginal discharge? Its timing associated with skin rash?*
- *Have you travelled abroad recently?*
- *Did insects bite you?*
- *Any possible exposure to industrial or domestic toxin?*
- *Any possible contact with venereal disease?*
- *Was there close physical contact with others that have skin disorders?*
- *Any possible exposure to HIV?*
- *Past history of skin problems. Is this the first time?*
- *Past Medical History*
- *Environmental and psychological factors*
- *Allergy, Meds*
- *Family history of skin and internal disease*

Physical Exam:

1. Inspection:
- Distribution and arrangement (annular, linear...), symmetry of lesions
- Lesion size, shape, location, configuration, pedunculation.
- Color of lesions, blanching
- Elevation or depression, swelling base
- Uniformity of lesions
- Thickness of skin

- Hygiene of skin, odors, presence of exudates
- Type: Papule (<1 cm raised), plaque >1 cm raised; macula (<1 cm flat), patch(>1cm flat) vesicle/bulla, pustule, erosion, ulcer, wheal, scar, crust, scale, fissure, excoriation, lichenification, xerosis, atrophy, comedones, petechia, purpura, ecchymosis.
- Remember to examine hair, mucous membrane and nails

2. Palpation:
Moisture, temperature, texture, turgor.

4. Joint Pain.

Case 1.
50 YOM complains of bilateral joint pain. History and physical exam in 10 minutes.

Case 2.
55 YOF complains of joint pain. Take a focus history and physical exam in 10 minutes.

Keys:
1. Are the patient's complaints truly articular or non-articular?
2. Is the arthritis inflammatory or degenerative?
3 Is the problem local or systemic?
4. How sick is the patient?

History:
General questions:
Age, occupation, past medical history, family history, medications, review of systems.

Specific questions:
OPQRST – *Onset, Precipitating/alleviating factors, Quality, Radiation, Site, Timing.*

* *Where is the maximal site of pain? Unilateral or bilateral?*
* *How long has she/he been having this problem? When did it start? Acute (hrs), subacute (days), insidious (months)?*
* *What else happens along with it?*
  – Inflammatory symptoms: morning stiffness, tenderness, swelling, redness, warmth
  – Mechanical/degenerative symptoms: worse at end of the day, better with rest; locking, give way, instability
  – Neoplastic and infectious symptoms: constant pain, occurs at night fever, night sweats, anorexia, fatigue, weight loss
  History of prostate, thyroid, breast, lung or kidney Ca-- "P.T. Barnum

Loves kids"
— Referred pain: shoulder pain from heart, arm pain from neck, leg pain from back
Then cardiac, GI, GU history, have to be obtained

- *Is there evidence of inflammation? Any swelling? Any fluid in the joint?*
- *Does the pain change during the course of the day? Any stiffness? Does pain get better or worse as you move? Does the knee lock at a certain position?*
- *How much does it affect your daily life? get up, use bathroom, comb hair, transfer from shower or tub, etc.*
- *Over the years, are there any changes to the severity of pain?*
  Intermittent with return to baseline
  Gradual progression with acute exacerbation
  Wax and wane with slow progression over time
- *Do you have problems with your (extra articular) skin, kidney, eyes, lung, GI*

- Characteristics of Pain:

	Inflammatory	Non-inflammatory
Morning stiffness	+>30min	-<30min
Worse after	rest	use
Signs of inflammation	rubor (red), tumor(swelling) calor (warm)	only tumor (swelling)
Instability	-	+

Physical Exam:

Key:
Always examine the joint above and below

- Look: shape, position
SEADS: Swelling, **E**rythema, muscle **A**trophy, **D**eformity, **S**kin changes
- Feel: temperature, tender, effusion, crepitus, laxity/instability, soft tissue, bursa.
- Move:

Active or passive range of motion (ROM), crepitus, abnormal
   mobility
Passive ROM>active ROM suggest soft tissue inflammation or
   muscle weakness
- Neurovascular:
   Pulse, reflex, power, sensation
   Special test: Lachlan's, McMurray's
- Observe gait:
   Walking, heel to toe, on heels, on toes
   Trendlenburg gait in hip disorders
   Antalgic, high stepping, circumduction

Investigation:
- Blood:
   General – CBC, lytes, BUN, Cr
   Acute phase reactants – ESR, C3, C4, fibrinogen, C-reactive
   protein, albumen
   Serology - RF, ANA, Ag-Ab complexes
- Synovial fluid:
   Gross appearance: volume, color, clarity, viscosity
   3Cs: cell count + differential, crystal, culture and sensitivity
- X-ray:
   Inflammatory-diffuse erosion
   Non-inflammatory-local cartilage loss, decreased joint space,
   bony overgrowth, erosion

Differential Diagnosis:
- Inflammatory articular:
   RA, SLE, scleroderma, psoriatic, Reiter's syndrome, anky
losing spondylitis, gout, gonacoccal, Lyme disease
- Non-inflammatory articular:
   Osteoarthritis, hypertrophic pulmonary osteoarthropathy,
   myxedema, amyloidosis.
- Inflammatory peri-articular:
   Polymyalgia rheumatica, dermatomyositis, eosinophilia-
   myalgia syndrome
- Non-inflammatory periarticular:

Fibromyalgia syndrome, reflex sympathetic dystrophy
- Differentiate articular from Nonarticular: location, aggravation/releasing factors, functional loss
- Differentiate inflammatory from non-inflammatory: redness, warmth, swelling, tenderness
- Specific etiology:

a. distribution and timing (acute/chronic)

b. severity

c. age and gender: ankylosing/RA - before 40 Y/O, SLE pre-menopausal women, gout-post menopausal, men all ages, SLE, RA - female, Reiter's - male

d. Associated Sx:
- Fever-infection, allergy, RA;
- RA-morning stiffness,
- OA-severe with use
- Rash-SLE, gonococcus, lyme, vasculitis
- Raynaud's – SLE, scleroderma, RA
- Diarrhea – inflamatory bowel disease
- Reiter's-conjunctivis, urethritis
- Fibromyalgia-sleep disorder, chronic fatigue
- Sjogren's-dry mouth, dry eyes

e. PMHx SHx FHx gout, STD, travel, tick bite

5. Hair and Nail Abnormality

Case 1.
45 YOM complains of hair loss, take a history in 5 minutes.

Case 2.
26 YOF complains of nail cracking, assess.

History for hair loss
* *Was the hair loss sudden or gradual?*
* *Does it occur only on scalp or body hair involved as well?*
* *Is the baldness localized or generalized? Symmetric or asymmetric?*
* *Is there family history of baldness?*
* *What drugs, meds have you taken recently?*
* *Any recent illness, stress, or trauma?*
* *Are there other systemic symptoms?*

Hair Assessment:
1. Inspection:
   Color, distribution, quantity, area of hair loss
2. Palpation for texture

Nails assessment:
1. Inspection:
   Pigmentation of nails and beds
   Length, symmetry
   Ridging, pitting, pealing
2. Measure nail base angle
   Clubbing
3. Nail folds:
   Redness, swelling, pain
   Exudates, warts, cysts, tumors

4. Nail plates:
   Texture, firmness
   Thickness, uniformity

Adherence to nail bed

Case 3.

46 YOF complains of hirsutism, take a history in 5 minutes.

History:

- *Any other family member with similar problems? (Familiy history)*
- *Is your menstrual period regular?*
- *Any history of primary or secondary infertility?*
- *Any history of visual disturbances or headaches (pituitary)?*
- *Meds: phenytoin, anabolic steroid, and progesterone.*

6. Weight Loss

Case 1.
66 YOM, complains of recent weight loss. Take a focus history in 5 minutes.

Key:
Try to find the cause, especially mention possible underlying malignancy.

History:
- *How much weight loss during what time span?*
- *Is the weight loss intentional?*
- *Do you enjoy your meals? Appetite?*
- *Can you describe your usual breakfast, lunch and supper? Eating habits and average daily diet?*
- *Does eating cause pain or any discomfort?*
- *Any nausea, vomiting, abdominal pain?*
- *Is your stool normal in color and consistency?*
- *Do you have fever, night sweats, tremor, and weather intolerance?*
- *Do you pass excessive volumes of urine?*
- *FHx, drinking history, smoking history, use of drugs.*
- *Any other illness, such as mass, pain, cough, etc? – R/o cancer*
- *Anything happened in your life, in your family? – Stress event*

7. Infertility

Case 1.
35 YOM, infertility, take a focused history in 5 minutes.

Key:
Focus on possible etiology, especially treatable causes.

History:
- *Have you or your partner ever conceived?*
- *Do you have difficulty obtaining or maintaining an erection?*
- *Do you ejaculate?*
- *Do you understand the timing of ovulation in your partner?*
- *Are you on any Meds that may cause impotence or sperm malformation (e.g. salazepyrine)*
- *Have you noticed any change in facial hair growth?*
- *Have you ever had cancer treatment – chemo, radiation?*
- *Have you had any operation in your groin? (Herniorrhaphy?)*
- *Have you had any operation on your testicles?*
- *Do you have: hypertension, peripheral vascular disease, diabetes, multiple sclerosis, spinal injuury?*
- *Are you overly stressed?*

8. Joint Exam

Hip
Inspection:
- Stance, swing, lumbar spine-lordosis, anterior-posterior of hip for muscle atrophy and bruising
- Gluteal fold, symmetry is important.

Palpation:
- Anterior-iliac crest, iliac tubercle, anterior superior iliac spine
- Posterior-superior iliac spine, great trochanter, trochanter bursa, ischial tuberosity, ischiogluteal bursa, sciatic nerve
- Front-Inguinal ligament-nerve, artery, vein, empty space, lymph node (NAVEL), below ligament-ilial psoas bursa

ROM:
- Shortening of one leg, measure length
- Abduction and flexion deformity
- Exaggerated lordosis
- Trendelenburg test: stand on affected leg, see if centralateral side drops or body leaning over supported leg
- Ortolani test: flex-abduct-touch table
- Barlow's sign: potential dislocate– Flex in/out

Knee
Inspection:
- Gait, alignment and contour, hollows around patella
- Genus valgum or varum
- Bulk of quadriceps muscle, measure diameter
- Effusion/swelling in joint

Palpation:
- Bone: medial/lateral femoral condyle, medial/lateral tibial plateau, patttela
- Muscle: quadriceps, patella tendon, medial/lateral ligament

- Meniscus and bursa-prepattellar bursa, anserine bursa, semimembranosus bursa
- Joint effusion-milk sign, balloon sign, bulge sign, balloting sign

ROM:
- Stability, Lachmann test, anterior/posterior drawer test, for checking the ligaments
- McMurray's test: internal/external rotations to test lateral/medial meniscus
- Remember to look at back of the joint

Shoulder
Inspection:
- Contour, effusion, deformity-dislocation, muscle atrophy (deltoid, peri-scapular, supra/infra spinus)

Palpation:
Bone:
  - Clavicular, scapular, humerus, great tubercle
  - 4 joints: SC, ST, AC, GH
Muscle:
  - Pectoris major and minor.
  - SITS– rotator culf, supra/infra spinus, teres minor, subscapularis
  - Axioscapular group– trapezius, rhomboids, serratus anterior and levator scapula
Bursa:
- Subacromial bursa
- Axillary nerve distribution

ROM:
- Flexion-Extension, External rotation-Internal rotation, Abduction-Adduction, touch opposite shoulder, dropping sign
- Cervical:
  Wing scapula-long thoracic nerve, muscle power

Elbow

Inspection:

- Alignment, swelling on either side of olecranon, olecranon bursa

Palpation:

- Rheumatoid nodule
- Tennis and golfer elbow
- Ulner nerve

ROM:

- Flexion-Extension, supination-pronation
- Muscle: biceps, bronchioradialis, triceps, supinator, pronator muscles

9. Visual Disturbances

Case 1.
70 YOM complains of visual disturbances or diplopia. Obtain a focused history in 5 minutes.

Key:
Two conditions require emergency measures (1) temporal arteritis, (2) cental retinal artery occlusion.

History:
General questions:
Age, occupation, past medical history, family history, medications, review of systems.

Specific questions:
Vision loss
- *Is the vision loss unilateral or bilateral?*
- *Is it confined to one area of the vision field?*
- *Are there positive as well as negative visual phenomenon?*
- *Does color appear different?*
- *History of trauma, headache?*
- *Timing of problem, sudden gradual, duration?*

Diplopia
- *Is the diplopia relived by covering one or other eye?*
- *Is it horizontal, vertical, or oblique?*
- *Does it getting worse in one particular direction of gaze?*
- *Does the diplopia fluctuate or is it constant?*

Others
- *Have you felt fatigued, unwell?*
- *Do you have sore joints?*
- *Do you have severe headaches?*
- *Have you had a fever or night seats?*
- *Have you lost weight?*
- *Have you had pain in your jaw when eating?*

10. Sore Throat

Case 1.

60 YOF complains of sore throat or sore mouth. Obtain a focus history in 5 minutes.

Key:

Have a differential diagnosis in mind when asking specific
  questions.

History:

General questions:

Age, occupation, past medical history, family history, medications, review of systems.

Specific questions:

- *How long have you had the pain?*
- *Does the pain change in severity?*
- *Anything makes it worse/better?*
- *Is the pain localized or diffuse?*
- *What other illness you have?*
- *What Meds are you taking?*
- *Do you smoke/drink? How many cigarettes a day? How much alcohol?*
- *Are you sexually active?*
- *Do you have unprotected sex?*

11. Deafness

Case 1.
51 YOM complains of deafness, obtain a focused history in 5 minutes.

Key:
You may actually speak to the accompanying family member because the patient cannot hear you. Remember to keep eye contact with the patient, not the family member.

History:
General questions:
Age, occupation, past medical history, family history, medications, review of systems.

Specific Questions:
- *Did this happen suddenly or gradually?*
- *Is it progressive or static? Notice any changes in symptom?*
- *Is it unilateral or bilateral?*
- *Are there any other family members having similar problem?*
- *Have you been exposed to excessive noise recently?*
- *Have you had an ear infection before? (Otitis Media)*
- *What antibiotic have you been given before?*

12. Lump in the Throat

Case 1.

58 YOF complains of feeling a lump in the throat. Obtain a focused history in 5 minutes.

Key:

You can only diagnose depression after ruling out other pathology.

History:

General questions:

Age, occupation, past medical history, family history, medications, review of systems.

Specific questions:

- *Onset, changes over time?*
- *Any trouble swallowing? (dysphagia)*
- *Is the action of swallowing painful? (odynophagia)*
- *Any night sweats, weight loss?*
- *Do you suffer from heartburn, indigestion, taste of acid in the mouth?*
- *Anything upsetting you recently?*

13. Blocked Nose

Case 1.
62 YOM complains of blocked nose. Obtain a focus history in 5 minutes.

Key:
Prolonged blockage in one side, need to rule out tumor.

History:
General questions:
Age, occupation, past medical history, family history, medications, review of systems.

Specific questions:
- *One side, or both sides?*
- *Blocked constantly or intermittently?*
- *Does it vary with season?*
- *Any nose discharge? Any blood in the discharge?*
- *Anything makes it worse or better?*
- *Do you use nose drops? What, how frequent, when started?*
- *Do you sniff glue of illicit substance (e.g. cocaine)?*
- *Have you had previous nose surgery?*
- *Do you suffer from asthma?*

14. Hoarseness

Case 1.
*55 YOM complains of coarse voice. Obtain a history in 5 minutes and pro-
vide a differential diagnosis in the next 5 minutes?*

Key:
Hoarseness for more than 2-3 wks requires an exam of the larynx
to rule out malignancy.

History:
General questions:
*Age, occupation, past medical history, family history, medications, review of
systems.*

Specific questions:
- *Onset sudden or gradual, Getting worse/better? Anthing makes it worse or
  better?*
- *Any previous URTI-fever, sore throat, malgia?*
- *Any recent endoscope? Anesthesia?*
- *Any weight loss, cough, neck mass, chest pain, hemoptysis?*-tumor
- *Any thyroid disease? Surgery?*
- *Have you abused your voice? ie. Shouting, singing, crying?*
- *Do you smoke? If so, how many a day?*
- *How much alcohol do you drink?*
- *What type of work do you do?* Exposure to dust, fumes
- *Pain in the throat? Any time of the day-worse?*
- *Pain in breathing, swallowing and talking?* Difficulty in breathing or
  stridor suggest obstruction indicate emergency.
- *Is hoarseness exacerbated by talking? If voice completely disappeared, if so
  for how long?*
- *Character of voice?*

Breathy voice – cord apposition due to tumor, polyp, nodule
Raspy voice – cord thickening, edema, or inflammation due to
  infection, chemical irritation, vocal abuse
High shaky voice, or very soft tone: trouble mounting adequate
  respiratory force

Differential Diagnosis:

Acute:
- Laryngitis: viral infection, vocal abuse, toxic fume, allergy
- Laryngeal edema: angioneurotic, infection, direct injury, nephritis, epiglottis

Chronic:
- Laryngitis: vocal abuse, smoking, allergy, persistent irritant exposure
- Carcinoma of the larynx
- Vocal cord lesion: polyps, leukoplakia, contact ulcer, granuloma, nodules, benign tumor
- Vocal paralysis: brain stem lesion, laryngeal nerve injury, aorta aneurysm, tumor, surgery
- Vocal cord trauma: chronic intubation
- Systemic: hypothyroidism, RA, virilization
- Psychogenic

Investigations:
- Laryngoscopy

15. Repeated Epistaxis and Skin Bruises

Case 1.

30 YOF with repeated epistaxis and skin bruises. Take a history and per-form a physical exam in 10 minutes. Which investigation does she need?

Keys:

1. If ecchymosis, occurs spontaneously on the trunk; >3 cm in diameter is worrisome.
2. First, check vitals to R/O serious hemorrhage or volume deple-tion.
3. ITP is often associated with lymphoma, CLL, HIV, connective tissue diseases, etc.

History:
General questions:
Age, occupation, past medical history, family history, medications, review of systems.

Specific questions:
* *Are you bleeding now? How much blood? Do you feel difficulty in breathing? Light headedness, marked fatigue?*
* *Onset, location, duration, and clinical course, precipitating factors?*
* *Spontaneous or traumatic? How frequent?*
* *Amount of bleeding? difficulty in stop bleeding? Nasal obstruction?*
* *Any treatment?*
* *Precipitating factors: URTI, dry heat, nose picking, forceful nose blowing?*
* *Associated Symptoms: pain, fever, weight loss, adenopathy, night sweating?*
* *Current illness: URTI; liver, kidney or bone marrow disease?*

Physical Exam:
Look for evidence of bleeding, look for hepatosplenomegaly.
* Vitals: check for significant volume depletion
* General appearance: Cushingnoid, Marfanoid

- Signs of systemic disease: septicemia, fever, toxic anemia, adenopathy, splenomegaly
- Skin and mucous membrane:
    a. size, number, location of bleeding. petechia <3cm, purpura <1cm, ecchymosis >3cm
    b. Spider nevi, teleangiectasia
    c. Vascular fragility test
- Systemic:
    Adenopathy, hepato-splenomegaly
    Joints and muscles for hematoma and hemoarthroses
- DRE: For evaluation of GI bleeding.

Investigation:
- CBC, blood smear, platelet count
- Bleeding time, PT, PTT, INR
- Platelet quality: aggregation test, ristocetin-induced agglutination
- Testing for cause of thrombocytopenia:
    1. Peripheral blood smear
    2. Bone marrow exam
    3. Platelet-bound IgG autoantibody
    4. HIV serology
- Other: LFTs, RFTs,FDP, ESR

Differential Diagnosis:
- Platelet:
  Qualitative platelet disorder: Von Willebrand's disease, NSAID
  Quantitative platelet disorder:
  (1). Increased destruction- ITP, TTP, vasculitis, drug, immune/non-immune,
  (2). Splenic sequestration, hypersplenism,
  (3). Decrease production – marrow disease, aplastic anemia, fibrosis, lymphoma/leukemia, myelodysplastic syndrome, multiple myeloma
- Coagulation factor
  Extrinsic: Vitamin K deficiency
  Intrinsic: Hemophilia A, B
- Vascular factor

Scurvy, Cushing's, drug-induced, hereditary, connective tissue
- Systemic: renal failure, liver failure, DIC, HIV

Investigations:
- CBC, blood smear
  – In ITP, HB and WBC normal, thrombocytopenia.
- BM aspiration/biopsy
  – In ITP filled with megakaryocytes
- Abdominal U/S
  – spleen size

Treatment of ITP:
1. Prednisone is the initial therapy in the most patients.
2. Platelets less than 10 000-20 000 with failure of medical therapy should undergo splenectomy
3. Intravenous immunoglobulin or Rhogam is used in the initial therapy of patients with profoundly low platelet counts <10 000 and life threatening bleeding
4. Platelet transfusions are almost never used except in life threatening bleeding in which steroid and Ig did not sufficiently correct the platelet count.

16. Dizziness and Vertigo

Case 1.
A man presents with a complaint of dizziness. Take a focused history in 5 minutes and provide a differential diagnosis in the next 5 minutes.

Key: Differentiate vertigo from non-vertigo, try to find etiology.

History:
General questions:
> *Age, occupation, past medical history, family history, medications, review of systems.*

Specific questions:
- *What do you mean by dizziness or vertigo?*
- *When started, how long did it last? Does it come and go?*
- *Do you feel lightheaded, confused? Or giddy or dazed?*
- *Is there an experience of rotation?*
- *Do you feel you are spinning or outside around you is spinning?*
- *Is the dizziness accompanied by unsteadiness when walking?*
- *Is it triggered only by a certain movements or head position, standing or turning?*
- *Is it getting worse when you close your eyes? Move your head? If yes = vestibular*
    1. True vertigo (vestibular; faintness)
    2. Postural (cardiovascular)
    3. Poor balance/multiple sensory deficits (cerebellar)
    4. Ill defined, light headed (psychotic)
- *Onset: When do you start to have this feeling? Anything happened at home, work. Were you sick?*
- *Duration:How long does it last?*
    1. Flash (Psychogenic)
    2. A minute (BPPV, vascular)
    3. Minutes to 24 hours (Menière's disease)
    4. Days (acute vestibular)
    5. Months to years (Psychogenic, CNS, multisensory loss)

- *Any Associated Symptoms?*
1. Neurologic: diplopia, dysphasia, ataxia, TIA, VBI, arrhythmia indicate central vertigo.
2. Auditory: hearing loss, tinnitus, otalgia, labyrinthitis, pressure in the ear, ototoxic drugs, indicate peripheral vertigo
3. Anti-HTN, tranquilizer, or anti-depressant toxicity: standing or turning causes light headedness
4. Non-specific: n/v
- *Using any drugs recently, especially gentamycin?*

Differential Diagnosis:
Vertigo (vestibular)
- **Central:** Brain stem, cerebellar caused by tumor, stroke, drugs.
- **Peripheral:** Inner ear, vestibular nerve, Meniere's, BPPV caused by tumor, trauma, drugs, and infection

Non-vertigo
- **Ocular:** Decreased visual acuity
- **Vascular:** VBI, TIA basilar migraine, orthostatic HTN, arrhythmia, CHF, aortic stenosis, stroke.
- **Metabolic:** Hypoxia, hypoglycemia, hyper- hypocapnia.
- **Psychiatric:** Anxiety, depression, psychosis

Physical Exam:
- Otoscopy, tuning fork tests
- Evaluation for Nystagmus
- Cranial nerves-especially cranial nerve V, include corneal reflex
- Long-tract signs: cerebellar, pyramidal, and sensory
- Fundoscopy
- Investigation:
- Audiometry, caloric testing
- Evoked potentials, ENG, CT/MRI

17. Headache

Case 1.

40 YOF with history of headache. Obtain a focused history and perform a physical exam in 10 minutes. List differential diagnosis and investigations in the next 5 minutes or provide a treatment plan.

Key

1. Beware of the warning signs such as new onset, sudden, worst headache ever, associated fever, projectile vomit, LOC deteriorate, neurology sign, head injury, optic disc edema.
2. For temporal arteritis, initiate steroid treatment immediately.

History:
Onset:
- *Is this something new? Or have you experienced a bad headache before, any difference between then and now?*
- *Age of onset? When started? Acute or chronic?*
- *Has anything happened at home, at work or physically that initiated the pain?*
- *Any trauma?*
- *When does your pain start? Early morning, during day, during night, gradual vs. abrupt?*

Location:
- *Where does it hurt the most? Entire head, unilateral or specific site*
- *Is it always in here?*

Duration:
- *How long does it last? Minutes, hours, days, weeks*
- *Any pain free periods? Does it occur in clusters?*

Character:
- *What is it like? Throbbing, pounding, constant pressure, worse with movement?*
- *How severe? Can you grade the pain from 1 to 10?*

Pattern:
- *Worse in the morning, or as day progresses or occurs only during sleep?*

- *Can you describe a typical episode? What happens before, during, after headache?*
- *Is there any change in the pattern?*
- *How frequent?*

Aggravating/Relieving Factors:
- *Notice any changes in the pattern of headache?*
- *What situation would incite headache or make it worse?*
- *What situation makes it better?*
- *Can it be relieved by medication, sleep, or just resolve spontaneously*
- *Does the pain radiate anywhere else?*

Associated Symptoms:
- *Do you have N/V, fever?*
- *Do you ever lose your conscious?*
- *Notice arms/legs for sensation or power change?*
- *Problems in sight or vision, hearing, smelling, eating (bite)? Discharge from nose/ear?*
- *Any lacrimation, photophobia, fever, neck stiffness, seizures?*

Precipitating factors:
- *Fever, fatigue, stress, food, alcohol, allergy, menstrual cycle*

PMHx:
- *Do you drink, smoke, taking Meds, using drugs?*
- *Any serious illness, admission before?*
- *Any head trauma, recent lumbar puncture, surgery, seizure*

SHx:
- *Employment: risk of head injury, use of helmet, exposure to toxins and chemicals*
- *Stress, tension, demands at home, work, school*
- *Potential risk of injury: participation in sports, not using seat belts, unsafe environment*
- *Nutrition: recent weight gain/loss, skipping meals*

FHx:
- *Any family member with similar problem? Which type or character*
- *Any family member with thyroid dysfuntion?*

Physical Exam:
- Vitals: BP, pulse rate (PR), respiratory rate (RR), temperature.

- Head: appearance, hair, skins, and scar, where hurts
- Vessel bruits carotid, temporal, occipital
- Temporal-mandibular joint (TMJ)
- Nose: discharge, frontal/maxillary sinus, translucent
- Ear: discharge, hearing, mastoid
- Eye: pupil, cornea clouding (glaucoma), visual, fundi, pressure
- Oral cavity: teeth, trigger points.
- Cranial nerve
- C-spine, rigidity
- Neurology sign: ataxia, assessment of LOC, deficits

Investigation:
- CBC, ESR, CSF, plain sinus film, CT, MRI, Temporal Artery-biopsy

Differential Diagnosis:
Chronic recurrent headache:
a. Muscle contraction
   Psychogenic-depression/anxiety/stress/tension
   Cervical osteoarthritis, TMJ disease
b. Vascular
   Migraine, cluster
c. Drugs
Acute headache:
a. Infectious-meningitis, encephalitis
b. Post-trauma-concussion, cerebral contusion, subdural/epidural hematoma
c. Vascular-subarachroid hemorrhage, intracerebral hemorrhage
d. Elevated ICP-space occupying lesion, malignant hypertension, benign intracranial HTN
e. Local: temporal arteritis, acute angle closure glaucoma
Intracranial: mass, cerebral vascular, migraine, meningitis, post-concussion
Extra cranial: tension, sinusitis, giant cell arteritis, TMJ, cluster, Indomethasin-Responsive, systemic infection/fever, HTN, ocular, cervical radiculopathy, trigeminal neuralgia

Treatment:

- Migraine:
  Prevent: remove precipitant, NSAID, physiotherapy, Verapamil (calcium channel blocker)
  Aura: aspirin, ergotamine
  Full blown: ergotamine, meperidine, antiemetic
- Tension headache: aspirin, NSAID, Physiotherapy, antidepressant
- Cluster headache: O2, ergotamine, NSAID, avoid alcohol, Verapamil, Prednisone
- Temporal arteritis: Start Prednisone 60 mg OD as soon as possible, otherwise he or she will become blind.

Case 2.

50 year old female with severe headache, left side scalp tenderness, loss of vision in left side from 2 hours ago for a few minutes, pain on chewing. Do a history and physical in 10 minutes and answer the following questions in the next 5 minutes.

History and physical exam: same as case 9.

Diagnosis: Temporal arteritis.

3 Investigations:

- Temporal artery biopsy, ESR, and arteriography.

Treatment:

- Steroid; 40-60mg/day until symptoms resolve, then gradual tapering.

18. AIDS, Physical Exam

Case 1.
A 35 YOM tested positive for HIV, assess.

Case 2.
a. HIV positive patient c/o tachypnea, PE
b. CXR bilateral interstitial marking, Dx, DDx, treatment
c. Interpret CXR: PCP, AIDS, dyspnea, consulting

Keys:
1. HIV and AIDS are not equivalent. Signs of infection or malignancy in HIV+ patient indicate the development of AIDS.
2. Be focused. Look for the specific signs described below.

PE:
General:
   Vitals and general appearance – fever, malnutrition, BP, dehydration
Skin and mucous membranes:
   • Kaposi's sarcoma
   • Morbiliform eruption
   • Seborrheic dermatitis
   • Eosinophilic pustular folliculitis
   • Herpes simplex/herpes zoster-nasolabial and genital areas/ chest wall
   • Warts – Molluscum contagiosum, HPV, hairy leukemia
   • Bacteria/fungal infection.
HEENT:
   • Sinus infection,
   • Eyes: CMV retinitis.
   • Oral cavity: Hairy leukoplakia, thrush, mucosal petechiae, stomatitis, gingivitis and kaposi sarcoma, angular cheilitis
LN: Persistent generalized lymphadenopathy

Heart:

Murmurs and rubs – pericarditis/myocarditis/endocarditis

Lung:

Pneumonia, PCP, pluritis

- While taking hx, talking, watch for respiratory distress and other pulmonary clues
- Clubbing, cyanosis (central, peripheral)
- CO_2 retention: tremor, headache, and warm periphery, bounding pulse
- JVP-cor pulmonae, CHF
- Chest:

Inspection: Chest wall deformity and inequality, pattern of breathing, rate, rhythm, depth.

Palpation: Trachea displacement; vocal fremitus; precardial pulsation; chest expansion

Percussion: In sequence, dullness, consolidation, pleural effusion/inflammation, Hyperresonance.

Ansculation: Vocal resonance, whisper pectoriloquy, added sounds.

- If appropriate, measure flow rate

Joint:

Arthritis, vasculitis, sensory/motor dysfunction

Neural:

Meningitis/encephalitis-meningeal irritation, focal defects

Mental status- dementia

Peripheral neuropathy/myopathy

Abdomen: liver, spleen, mass, tender

GU: DRE, Pap smear, and lesion

Dx:

Pneumocystis Carinii Pneumonia

DDx:

Tuberculosis, Mycobacterium Avium intracellulare Pneumonia, CMV

Describe findings on CXR

Treatment:
– Oxygen: Keep SO2>90%
– Septra (SMX+TMP)
– Pentamidine aerosol
– Treat HIV: 3TC, AZT. IDV

PCP: Abrupt onset, high fever, tachypnea, nonproductive cough, and cyanosis. Pulmonary findings may be slight and disproportionate to the degree of illness and to the radiology findings. CXR: interstitial pattern (but may see heterogeneous distribution of infiltrate, diffuse or focal consolidation, cystic changes, nodules or cavitations)

19. Ankle Edema

Case 1.

30 YOM presented with bilateral ankle edema and pain after canoeing, do a focused history. 5 min.

Case 2.

30 YOM has pitting edema/ SOB for 1 month, He is on lasix for the last month, Do physical exam. 10 min.

Case 3.

27 YOM. swelling of ankles, no pain, no stiffness, Do Hx, Dx, Investigation and management.

Key:

History should reflect differential diagnosis.

DDx:

Unilateral

A. Hydrostatic pressure: deep vein thrombophlebitis, venous insufficiency

B. Capillary permeability: cellulitis, trauma

C. Lymphatic obstruction

Bilateral

A. Oncotic pressure: malnutrition, liver failure, nephrotic syndrome, protein-losing enteropathy

B. Hydrostatic pressure: CHF, RF, venous insufficiency, pregnancy, menstruation

C. Capillary permeability: systemic vasculitis, idiopathic edema, allergy

D. Lymphatic obstruction (retroperitoneal, or general)

E. Endocrine: Myxedema, Graves disease

F. Iatrogenic: MAO-inhibitor, anti-hypertensives, corticosteroids, estrogen, Progesterone, NSAIDS

G. Tauma

History

When did you start to notice the leg edema?
Is it one side, or both sides? Gradual or sudden onset?
Any changes during the day? Morning/afternoon better
Palliating (rest, elevation) and exacerbating factors?
Previous similar episodes, and lasted for how long?
Claudication symptoms? (Calf pain, relief with rest, reproducible)
Duration of canoeing prior to symptoms?

If one side:
Did you hurt yourself? Any redness, pain, Fever?
Recent surgery? Previous varicose, phlebitis?DVT?
Any joint problems?
Leg pain, parasthesia, weakness, loss of function?

If both sides:
How do you feel when the weather is turning cold? – thyroid
Do you have SOB? chest pain?
Do you jaundice, indigestion, bleeding problems – liver?
*Do you have hematuria, proteinuria, facial swelling, eyelid swelling, recent
    sore throat? – Kidney*
Do you have diarrhea, malabsorption? – GI
What Meds are you taking? Any new medications? Are you taking BCP?
Any allergy?

Physical exam:

If both sides:
Inspection: General appearance cachexia
    Face: jaundice, eyelid swelling
    Skin: color, cyanosis, spider nevi, bruising
    Neck: thyroid mass, JVP
    Chest: symmetry, shape, gynecomastia
    Abdomen: shape, ascites, scar, varicose
    GU: genital swelling
    Extremity: microcirculation, edema, lymph nodes, varicose,
    deep vein insufficiency
Palpation: thyroid, lymph nodes, pain, mass, hepatic-jugular reflux

Percussion: Hear, lung, liver, CVA, ascites, pleural effusion

Auscultation: heart (3rd sound), lung, thyroid, renal artery, bowel sounds

Edema: detail extent, calf and thigh diameter, compare both sides

If one side:

Tender, red, varicose, thrombosed vein (Homan's sign), pitting

Investigation:

If one leg:

Venogram, Doppler U/S, Impedance plethysmography, fibrinogen uptake, and lymphangiography

If both sides:

CBC lytes BUN Cr, CXR, Urine analysis, LFTs, TSH, GI work up, Throat swab, ASO, ANA, RF, compliment

Management

- Restrict salt intake (3g Na), normal protein 1g/kg/day, low Na (<1g/day)
- Avoid prolonged standing, sitting, elevate leg
- Support stocking
- Avoid salt-retaining drugs
- Diuretics
- Assure this condition is not a threat to health may be spontaneously subside
- Heparin for DVT
- Prednisone 1mg/kg x4-8 weeks for minimal change kidney disease,
- Treat etiology

Case 4.

In the post-exam (PEP) station:

- **Dx:** Nephrotic syndrome from minimal change glomerular nephritis.

- Tests: Urine micro, 24 hr urine protein, lytes, BUN, Cr, serum cholesterol and lipids, glucose, serum protein and albumin, Throat swab, ASO titer, ANA.
- Manage: Low salt high protein diet

Prednisone 60-mg PO

20. Drug Seeker

Case

20 YOM, from Saskatchewan, came here on business. He wants Fiorinal for tension headache. Says he only takes them irregularly. Very demanding and agitated.

Key:

Gentle consult, but be firm, do not give out a prescription.

Evaluation:

Are you having a headache now?
How frequent/severe you will have a headache?
Can you describe a typical pattern of headache?
How do you know headache is coming?
What happens when it comes? or when the pain starts going away?
Any N/V, Double vision, blindness or seeing stars?
Any previous investigation for the cause of it?
When have you had your last prescription?
Do you have the bottle with you?

– Education:

Fiorinal is a combination of analgesic/sedative drug (Fiorecet) consists of Acetaminophen or aspirin, butalbital, caffeine. Taking them can make you feel good, with a sense of increased energy and confidence. But if you take them frequently in high dose, it can cause serious health problems include tachycardia, fever, interstitial nephritis, etc. Prevously the drug contained phenacetin.

For patients with occasional headache like you, its better to establish an effective abortive regimen, avoid regular use. Stay away from it.

If bottles shows prescription recently and consume large dose, education is even more important.

21. Hand Weakness

Case 1.
Older man c/o right hand weakness, Hx, DDx, Dx, Investigation

Case 2:
24 YOM with transient left arm weakness and decreased vision. Hx, DDx, work up, immediate therapy.

Keys:
- Systemic disease vs. pathology of local structures.
- If sensation normal + proximal symmetrical pattern– indicate muscle disease
- If distal, non-symmetrical plus sensational abnormality-indicate nerve disease

History
Muscle weakness
- *Onset: When did you start to notice hand weakness? Is it sudden or gradual? In the morning or after activity?*
- *Any associated or causitive factors you can think of?*
- *Is the weakness global or focal? Is it symmetrical?*
- *Is it predominantly proximal or distal?*
- *Is the weakness secondary to pain?*
- *Is the weakness associated with sensory symptom such as numbness?*
- *Does the weakness fluctuate, static, or progressive?*
- *Is the weakness accompanied by feelings of stiffness or is the affected limb floppy?*
- *Is the weakness increasing in severity?*
- *Is there a FHx of muscle disease?*
- *Other problems with arm, leg, facial expression, vision, gait change?*
- *Any recent trauma, infection, fever, weight loss?*
- *PMHx: HTN, diabetes, heart, CVD, CAD, neurology, psychotic, seizure, AMPLE, stroke*

Weakness of the hand
- *Is the weakness associated with joint pain?*

- *Is it confined to the muscles supplied by a specific nerve (median, ulnar, radial)?*
- *Both hands involved or just one hand? Hand dominance?*
- *Is there accompanying sensory loss?*

If suspect a stroke
Where carotid/vertibrobasiler?
What ischemic/hemmorrhagic?
Why arthroscleorotic/embolic?

DDx
Neurological: central-stroke, peripheral-disk, C-spine, carpal tunnel
Vascular: claudication, thoracic outlet Syndrome
Muscular: trauma, Duchine myopathy
Endocrine: Myasthenia, hypothyroidism, Cushings
Metabolic: hypo- Na^+, Ca^{2+}
Tumor
Connective tissue: polymyocytis, dermatomyocitis

Investigation
Blood: CBC, lytes, PTT INR, VDRL, glucose, lipids
X-ray: C-spine, arm, CT MRI
Nerve conduction: electromyography
Vessel: Doppler, angiography -carotid
Cardiac: ECG, echocardiogram
Muscle enzyme:, EMG, muscle biopsy

Management:
– According to the etiology
For TIA: Modify risk factors; anti-platelets, ASA, Carotid endocarterectomy
For cerebral infarction: Prevent recurrence, death and complication
  ABCs, hydration, NPO, prevent DVT, alert MI, pneumonia, PE
  Avoid lower BP, high glucose

22. Dysphagia

Case
60 YOF, complains of dysphagia, Hx, investigation and treatment.

Keys:
Functional versus structural.
Esophageal versus non-esophageal

Hx:
- *What do you mean by dysphagia?*
  Can you take food by mouth? Are you having pain or are you having difficulty to swallow?
- *Does food move to the back of the oral cavity? ie., Can a swallow be initiated?*
- *Are you aware of the movement of food into your chest and abdomen?*
- *Do you feel food "sticking"? At what level?*
- *Are both food and drink equally difficult to swallow?*
  Any differences between hot/cold, bolus/non-bolus?
- *Is regurgitation associated with swallowing? Instant-oropharyngeal, intermittent-GERD, stricture*
- *Is there hx of reflux symptom like water brush, heart burn?*
- *Does the neck gurgle or bulge on drinking?*
- *Do you feel a lump in the throat all the time? globus hystericus*
- *When does this start? Is it happens suddenly or gradually?*
- *Any changes in Sx? Anything make the Sx work/better? Is it intermittent or progressive?*
- *Any mood changes? Do you feel depressed or anxious?*
- *Do you smoke, drink, using drugs, taking any Meds?*
- *Are you generally well, any serious disease? Chest pain, back pain, Weight loss?*
- *Do you ever have respiratory Symptom such as pneumonia, asthma (aspiration)? How frequent?*
- *Do you have bad breath at times? Or hear any complains about your bad breath?*   Halitosis – Zenkers diverticulum
- *Do you have thyroid disease/treatment? Any voice change, coughing, bone*

pain headache?

DDx:
- Oral cavity: viral ulcer, trauma, tumor, infection (Ludwig's angina)
- Oropharynx: tonsil, retropharyngeal abscess
- Hypopharynx: trauma, thyroid tumor, foreign body, inflammation, neuromuscular
- Esophageal:
a. Trauma/perforation
b. Obstruction
   Intrinsic: hiatal hernia, tumor, corrosive esophagitis/stricture, esophageal web, foreign body, diverticulum
   Extrinsic: mediastinal abnormality, vascular compression
c. Motility: achalasia, diffuse esophageal spasm, scleroderma, diabetic neuropathy

From Hx:
- Liquids + solids – achalasia
- Solids, intermittent – diffuse esophagal spasm – with chest pain, elderly patient
- Anxiety, young patient – lower esophageal ring
- Solids, progressive – with weight loss + odynophagia – carcinoma
- Chronic heart burn – peptic stricture

From Barium Swallow:
- Peptic esophagitis – prominent mucosa folds in distal esophagus
- Peptic stricture – smooth tapered narrowing
- Diffuse spasm – static contractile areas, poor propulsion or lodging of solid food bolus
- Carcinoma – abrupt narrowing, sharp angulation of margins
- Collagen disease – barium remains long after swallow, scleroderma
- Achalasia– dilated, tortuous, poor emptying, birds beak
- Diverticulum – typical protruding pouch

Investigation

PE-mouth, pharynx, neck
Barium swallow
Endoscopy + biopsy
Manometry
Provocative testing: acid perfusion-Bernstein test; Edrophonium
  testing
24 hr esophageal PH and pressure monitoring
Bronchoscopy, mediastinoscopy
CT

Manage

Motility Disorder:
Achalasia:
- Eating slowly, drinking small quantities at a time, avoiding cold
  foods
- A trial of sublingual nitrates or calcium channel blockers
- Anti-reflux therapy
- Anti-depressants, relaxation techniques and behavioral methods
- Esophageal dilatation, myotomy

Obstructive Disorder
- Dilatation
- Surgery
- Radiation/chemo
- Nutrition

Infection
- Anti-bacteria, anti-virus, anti-fungal

23. Alcoholic, Consult

Case 1.
Alcoholic caught drunk driving, wants help. Hx and consult.

Case 2.
A fit, healthy male needs counselling for alcoholic rehabilitation.

Key:
First assess drinking profile, amount, dependent,
  withdraw/addiction, tolerance, then provide medical consult

History
• Assess drinking profile
Usually at what time, where, on what occasion do you drink?
Anybody drink with you?
*How frequent? How many (bottle of beers, ounce of wine) do you drink in a
  week?*
Do you want to drink each time? Or do you have to drink?
*Has your drinking habit caused you any trouble at home, work or
  social relationship?*
Issues:
1) How are things going at home, work?
2) Safety issues, accidents, arrest, driving, depression (suicide intension)
3) Mood, why do you want to drink?

• Detection of alcohol abuse screening questions
 CAGE, HALT, BUMP, FATAL, DT
Cut down, Annoyed, Guilty, Eye opener
Drink to get high, drink Alone, Looking forward to drink, Tolerant
Blackout, Unplanned drinking, drink for Medical use, Protected supply
Family history, member of Anonymous, Think you self an alcoholic,
  Attempted suicide, Legal problems due to alcohol
Drive while intoxicated, use of Tranquilizer to steady your nerve

- **Be aware of alcohol-related medical problems**

GI: bleeds, liver disease, pancreatitis, oro/esophageal Ca
Heart: cardiomyopathy
Neurologic: double vision, nystagmous, gait, forget ness (Wernicke/Korsakoff)
Hematological: anemia, coagulopathy

- **Be aware of alcohol withdraw Sx**

Mild: 6-8 hr after, generalized anxiety, agitate, tremor, insomnia, N/V
Hallucination: 24-36-hr. visual/auditory
Seizure: generalized tonic-clonic
Delirium tremens: 3-5 days after, severe confusion, hyperpyrexia, diaphoresis,
  agitation, insomnia, hallucination/delusion, tremor, tachycardia

Consult
- Review the detrimental effect of alcohol on health, relationships, occupation, etc
- Address the fears and concerns of treatment, tough love technique. Keep motivation high, not only use patient's fear of losing something or someone important, but by getting him to seek and define his own reinforces
- Help patient identify, objectify and deal with anger and other emotions to enhance emotional control. Learn alternative ways of coping with people, situations associated with heavy drinking
- When patient ready, Provide information, appointment, and treatment modalities
a. Drug: For dependent – antabuse (disulfiram). For withdrawal – bezodiazepine, beta-blocker, thiamine
b. Treat on inpatient/outpatient bases.
c. Alcoholic anonymous
d. Psychotherapy, behavior approach, social and community help
- Encourage self-monitoring
- Involvement of family or significant others

24. Risks of HIV for Health Care Workers

Case 1
Nurse sustained needle stick injury. The patient is HBSAg+, HIV-, Advise and Manage.

Case 2.
A nurse who is going to work in the OR, concerned about risks of needle stick and related infection, Consult.

History
Where, when, what has happened?
Any other contact? Feces, urine, saliva
Are universal precautions taken: gowning, gloving, double bagging
Have you had a Hepatitis B vaccination? How many shots? Titer checked?

Consultation
- A needle stick increases the risk of getting Hepatitis by 20% (6-30%). This is why we all need to be vaccinated. If you are vaccinated, have your titer checked. You don't need to be treated. We can monitor your health at 0, 3, 6 month intervals.
- Possibility of getting HIV by a needle stick is 0.3%. There is no vaccine available, however, taking Zidovudine has been shown to reduce the risk of transmission by 80%.
- Universal precausion is very important.
- Also, we should emphasize the importance of safer sex.

Management
- Patient Hep B +, and you are vaccinated, no treatment. We can monitor you for 3-6 months.
 If you are not vaccinated, give HBIg 0.06 ml/kg immediately, Start vaccine 0,1,6 month, then monitor 0, 3, 6 months. Give within 14 days better, 30 days still effective
- Patient HIV +, combined therapy should start ASAP
 3TC 150mg bid x4wks
 AZT 200mg tid x4 wks

Indinavir (IDV) 800 tid x4wks
Monitor: 0, 3, 6, 12 months
• Patient HIV neg, still a small risk of HIV infection, he may be in the incubation period after recent HIV exposure. Advise using barrier method during sex for now. F/U with HIV test in 3-6 months time.

If stick, what can be done, what type of test/sensitivity of test, What will I tell my husband? Sex protection

Incidence of infection in North American
Hep. B-10%, HIV-no reliable estimate

HIV infection prevalence
1. Homosexual + bisexual male – 20-50%
2. IV drug users – 5-60%
3. Civilian applicants for military service 0.15%
4. Geography age, sex, ethnic background.

High risk groups for HIV and HBV
1. Homosexual and bisexual men
2. IV drug users
3. Person from endemic areas
4. Blood transfusion recipients or exposed to blood products (HIV 1977-1985 only)
5. Sexual partners of infected person
6. Children born to infected mother
7. Sexually activate person with many partners
8. Person with tattoos
9. Hx of Hepatitis, institutionalized-HBV only

Modes of transmission
1.Sexual contact
2.Needle stick
3. Breaks in skin
4. Splashes of blood or body fluid that contact mucous membranes, eye, mouth

5. Mother to child in uterus or during birth

All health care workers should consider blood/and body fluids of every patient as potentially infectious

Procedures to follow

1. Handle sharps, objects, and equipment with care
2. Don't recap, bend, break, or remove needles from syringe
3. Discard disposable needles/syringes, scalpels in furniture resistant containers located close
4. Specimen-collection protocol should be observed
5. Gloves should be worn when in contact with blood or body fluids or broken skin or mucous membrane
6. Change gloves after contact with each patient.
7. Wash hand after contact with blood/body fluids
8. Protective clothing i.e. Gowns, goggles, mask
9. In case of needle stick injury, report to health office and complete accident forms and protocal.

25. Fatigue

Case.

Male, c/o fatigue, Hx, DDx, Manage.

Key:

Try to find the etiology and manage accordingly.

Hx:

- *What do you mean by fatigue? Do you feel tired all the time? Pain anywhere?*
- *When you started feel fatigue? Was anything happening at home (any death? Relationship change, financial difficulty), at work? Were you sick? (> 3months+stresser, Psychogenic)*
- *Notice any changes in Sx? What makes you feel better? Rest/exercise? When do you feel better? Morning/afternoon*
- *Do you feel unable to do things or just don't want to do things?*
- *Can you complete half of you previous work?*
- *What about your sleep? Difficult fall asleep/early wake up, any snoring/sleep apnea, any food reflux when you lie flat?*
- *What about your appetite? Notice any weight loss?*
- *Do you have fever? Night sweats? Adenopathy?*
- *Any changes in bowel movement, urine frequency, heat/cold tolerance?*
- *Any mood change? Ever think of killing your self?*
- *Do you have any serous disease such as diabetes, SOB, HTN, liver, kidney disease, joint/bone pain?*
- *Are you on any Meds?*
- *Do you drink, smoke, and use drugs?*
- *What about the family situation? Good support or chaotic.*

DDx

a. Psychogenic: depression, anxiety, somatization disorder, personality, and eating disorder

b. Pharmacology: hypnotic, anti-HTNs, anti-depressants, tranquilizers, street drugs

c. Endocrine: diabetes, hypothyroidism, pituitary insufficiency, Addison's disease, renal/liver failure
d. Malignancy, anemia
e. Infection: endocarditis, TB, HIV
f. Cardiac/pulmonary failure
g. Connective tissue disease: RA
h. Disturbed sleep: sleep apnea, GE reflux, allergic rhinitis
i. Myasthesia gravis

Diagnosis

Chronic Fatigue Syndrome: New onset of persisting, relapsing or debilitating fatigue that impairs daily activities to or >50% of premorbid levels for at least 6 month; R/O physical signs/symptoms of psychological conditions

Manage

- Investigation: CBC lytes, ESR, Glucose, TSH, Urine analysis CXR EKG,
  Serology: EBV, CMV HIV, HBsAg, VDRL
- Treat etiology
- Undetermined etiology: reassurance, F/U, exercise, behavior/group therapy, vitamins
- Chronic fatigue syndrome: low dose anti-depressant, NSAIDs

26. Neck Pain and Back Pain

Case 1.
Man c/o neck pain, Hx. PE, DDx, Manage

Case 2.
70 YOF with neck pain and weakness in the left arm, focused exam.
Found: limited neck movements, mild weakness, abnormal sensation at thumb and 2nd fingers.
X-ray: narrowing of C6-7 disk space, describe, Dx and Tx.

Case 3.
32 YOM, had back pain for 1 year. Now the pain has become severe and radiates to the left leg. Do relevant back exam and focused Hx.
The examiner ask: Q: What is your diagnosis: Disk displaced.
Q: What is the level? L.5

Case 4.
45 yr, injured back 2 wks ago, treated by Tylenol #3 + beds rest, Now back pain more severe. Need to elicit trauma detail.

Keys
Red flags: Hx of trauma, hx of Ca, constitutional sx, IV drug use, chronic disease, age >50, neuromotor deficits, pain unrelieved, fever, sweats, chills, weight loss, bowel/bladder dysfuntion, saddle anesthesia.

History
• *Onset: Is the pain begins suddenly or gradually?*
  What happened? Any trauma or other particular cause you can think of?
  Trauma detail: How did you hurt your back? Did you hear a loud noise? Were you able to walk home?
• *Location: Where it hurts the most? Is the pain confined to the back or does it radiate to the upper or lower limb?*
• *What is the pain like? Aching, throbbing, cutting? How bad is it?*

- *Do you notice any change in severity? Anything make the pain worse/ better?*
  Which position/ situation (coughing) make it worse/ better?
  Does coughing or sneezing exacerbate the pain?
  Is it getting worse while walking but getting better while sitting/ bending--- spinal stenosis
  Is it getting worse while sitting, driving or lifting? – herniated disk
- *Do you feel numness or weakness in arm, legs?*
- *Do you have fever, weight loss? – malignancy such as multiple myeloma*
- *Do you have morning stiffness – ankylosing spondylitis*
- *Do you have any difficulty in controlling your bowel movement or bladder?*
- *AMPLE: Do you have coronary artery disease, angina? Meningitis N/V? Previous back surgery?*
- *Have you ever had a lumbar puncture? Current infection? Using high dose steroids?*
- *Past Hx of similar problems? Previous therapeutic efforts?*
- *Social Hx: Any problems at home, work? Under any stress? Financial problems?*
  Compensation issue?
- *FHx: Any family member/ close relatives had back problems*

PE:

Patient standing

a. Inspect-protruding abdomen, hyperlordosis, loss of lordosis, scoliosis, kyphosis
b. Gait, walk on heels (L4-L5) and toes (S1)
c. Squat L2,3,4
d. ROM-spine flexion-extension, internal/external rotation, side
e. Palpate: spinal, paraspinal and pelvic structures
f. Occiput to wall distance, chest expansion

Patient sitting

a. Straight leg raise (sciatica), flex knee then straighten to 90 degrees
b. Knee (L4) and ankle (S1) reflex
c Costal vertebrae angle (CVA)

Patient supine

a. Abdominal exam-IPPA

b. Vascular exam-pulse of femoral, popliteal, dorsalis pedis and posterior tibia

size, symmetry, swelling, pigmentation, ulcers

inguinal nodes, edema

raise both feet to 60 degrees, when pale, sit up and dangle feet

c. Sensory-light touch, pin prick

       L4-anterior medial thigh and knee

       L5-lat leg, web space

       S1-lat heel foot and toe

d. Motor-passive and resistance

       L4-quads, extend knee against resistance

       L5-dorsiflex great toe

       S1-plantar flex foot

e. Sacroiliac-compression test

f. Hip: ROM and Faber test for sacroiliac joint. Foot on opposite knee, press on knee

Patient prone

a. Sensory-S2-S4, anal wink-ask examiner for result

b. Sphincter tone-ask examiner for result

c. Femoral stretch-L2,4, hip and knee in extension

d. Motor exam-S1-gluteous maximus, backward lift leg against resistance

	Movement	Sensory	Reflex
C5	Deltoid	axillary	Middle Deltoid, bicep
C6	Bicep	1, 2 finger	Brachial-radialis, bicep
C7	Tricep	3 finger	Tricep
C8	Digital	4, 5 finger	Finger jerk

Investigation

X-ray film

CT/MRI

Bone radionuclide scans

Myelography

EMG

Immunoelectrophoresis

Management neck pain
Cervical Collar
Muscle relaxants
Non-narcotic analgesics
Home cervical traction
Spinal manipulation U/S diathermy
Surgery referral

Management back pain
- Bed rest (<4day) and analgesics, muscle relaxants, NSAIDs
- Activity: herniated disk: first week, walk 20 minutes 3x/day interspersed with bed rest
  adjust according to Sx; gradual increase
  Exercise and back care program
- Physiotherapy and spinal manipulation
- Surgery. Indications:
  1. Persistent disabling root pain despite 4-6 wks comprehensive conservative therapy
  2. Progressive neurologic deficits in the lower extremities
  3. Disruption of bowel/bladder control

DDx:
A: Surgical:
  a. Mild: muscle strain, ligament sprain, facet syndesis, degenerative disease, spondylolisthesis
  b. Moderate: sciatica – herniated disc, spinal stenosis
  c: Emergency: Cauda Equina syndrome-disc, mass, abscess, aorta aneurysm

B: Medical:
  a. Neoplasm – multiple myeloma, osteoid osteoma
  b. Infectious – acute discitis, osteomyelitis, TB
  c. Inflammatory – ankylosing spondylitis, psoriatic spondylitis, reactive arthritis, IBD
  d. Metabolic – osteoporosis, osteomalacia, paget disease

e. Viscera – endometriosis, pyelonephritis, pancreatitis, AAA

For low back pain
– With sciatica:
 Disc herniation; spinal stenosis; compression fracture; epidural abscess; intraspinal tumor/metastasis; vertebral osteomyelitis with compression fracture (late)
– Without sciatica:
 Musculoligmentous; ankylosing spondylitis; spondylolisthesis, depression; vertebral osteomyelitis (early); epidural abscess (very early); retroperitoneal neoplasm

Case 5.
A patient diagnosed with ankylosing spondylitis. Do Hx and PE in 10 minutes

Keys:
• Focus on issues that are specific for AS, such as FHx, age, progression, uveitis, aortitis, effects on breathing (chest expansion).

Hx:
See above, but focus on
• *Is it worse in the morning or later in the day? Morning stiffnes?*
• *How do you sleep? gesture*
• *Systemic:*
Any fever/chills, night sweats/wt loss, nocturnal pain, anorexia?
Ocular: Any symptoms of conjunctivitis? iritis? Uveitis?
CVS: Any chest pain, palpitation? Aortitis, aortic regurgitation
Cutaneous: Any skin rashes, mouth ulcers?
GI: Any diarrhea, abd pain?
GU: Any dysuria-urethritis? IgG nephropathy, amyloidosis?
MSK: Any other joint pain? Involve asymmetric large joint, often lower limb
 Any enthesitis dactylitis, Achilles' tendenitis
Other: Any adenopathy?
• *PMHx -malignacy, infections (TB), IV drug abuse, recent GU procedures, metabolic bone disease (menopause, anorexia nervosa, steroids)*
• *FHx: HLA B27 association*

PE:

See above but focus on

Spine: Occiput to wall distance, chest expansion, thoracic
   kyphosis, lumbar lordosis loss, ROM

Joint: asymetric large joint, lower extremity, SI joint

Eye, finger, Achilles tendon

Investigation:

X-ray: Bamboo spine; widening of SI joint, square lumbar spine

ESR, RF: Negative

27. Obesity

Case.
35 YOM previous healthy except obesity, interested in losing weight, consult.

Keys:
- Explore motivations.
- Provide information about consequences of obesity (health and psychosocial well being) and nutrition
- Set realistic goals.
- Offer support/reinforcement throughout the weight-losing process.

Approach:
1. Diagnosis
- Complete diet history
- Assess body mass index $= kg/m^2$
- Assess patients self-image: feel under/over weight or normal?
- Screen for eating disorder
- Personal/FMHx of obesity and nutrition problems

2. Manage:
- Discuss nutrition related problems
- Use Canada Food guide
- Discuss diet: FAD diet has no long-term benefit.
- There is no ideal weight, but rather a range of healthy weights
- Behavior modification: daily records of food eaten, eat slower and less, change envioronment and preparation style
- Exercise
- Group support
- Surgery

Hx:
- *Hello Mr…, I am Dr X, I understand that you are trying to lose some weight. Is that right?*
  Can you tell me why you are interested in losing weight at this point? Self-

image, health concerns?
- *How long have you been overweight? How much do you weigh? Your highest/lowest weight?*
- *Do you have- HTN, snoring, diabetes, joint degenerative disease? Notice anything abnormal other than obese: fatigue, voice change, skin/hair change, cold intolerance? edema, joint pain?*
- *How many meals do you eat per day, include snacks?*
  What do you eat each day? How much fat, fruit? Vegetables, bread?
  Do you eat while watching TV?
  Do you eat before going to bed?
  Do you have breakfast every day?
  Have you ever eat to calm down your nervous stomach?
  What do you think is wrong with your current diet?
- *What habit do you have? How much exercise do you do each week?*
- *Have you tried any program to lose weight? Does it work? Why stop?*
- *Is your family supportive about you losing weight?*

Consult

- *Now why are some people larger than others? Certainly there are genetic factors that we couldn't do anything about it. What we could do are two main things: modify our diet and exercise. In some people their weight problem is because of underlying disease, for you it is not the case.*
- Your ideal body weight is (M:106 1b for 5 Ft. + 6 lb/inch; F:100 lb/5Ft+5 lb/inch)
  >20% ideal weight is obesity
  Overweight increases the risks of HTN, CVD, CAD, Gall bladder disease, Fatty liver, diabetes, Cancer of breast, bowel, cervix, OA, obstructive sleep apnea, spinal dysfunction
- Diet:
  a. Your ideal calorie intake should be: ideal weight x10 Calorie (K)
  To lose 1 lb/ wk, should take 300-500k less
  1g fat-9k 1g carb-4k, 1g protein-4k
  b. Recommend bread, starch, fruit, vegetable, fish
  Avoid: cheese, fat, alcohol
  c. Diet medications such as FAD diet, not only no long-term benefit, they may even be dangerous for your health

- Behavior:
  Keep a record of food intake
  Eat only in one place, using smaller plate
  Prohibit another activity while eating
  Planning meals by shopping from list
  Having low calorie food available all the time
  Strategy for party: position away from food table
- Exercise:
  Begin with walk, specific time each day
  Regularly 30 min, 4-5 times per week
  Reach 60-80% maximum HR (200-age)
  Self monitoring, group
- Other: surgery, weight losing program/group
- *Lets plan to lose 1 lb next week by modifying food intake, I want you come back at the same time next week with a 3 day diary and another plan*

<u>1st visit:</u>
Orientation of patient to weight loss program
Examine current eating pattern (food diary)
Complete Hx and PE: Age of onset of obesity
   Number of previous attempts, how successful
   Present motivation
   Take weight
<u>2nd visit</u>
Review of weight, food diary (what, when and with whom food taken)
<u>3rd visit</u>
Review food dairy, weight, positive reinforcement of weight loss achieved, discuss if not achieved.

<u>4th and subsequent visit</u>
Review dairy, wt, and exercise precipitation, once weight down, reduce visit frequency F/U 6-12 month to assess continue adherence to the program.

28. Smoking Cessation

Case.
50 YOM, heavy smoker, consult regarding smoking cessation.

1st Visit
Scenario A:

Dr. *How many years have you been smoking? How many cigarettes a day? Are you interested in stopping smoking?*

Pt. *No, or not now.*

Dr. *Is there a special reason that you can't stop or don't want to stop?*

Pt: *Withdrawal, weight gain, other smokers, etc*

Dr. *Well, I respect your decision, but as you know, smoking causes many diseases, like lung Ca, CAD. It also affect the health of other people, for an example, passive smoking by your wife and children living in the same house. As a physician, I am concerned about your health and advise you stop smoking ASAP*

Dr. *Think about it, OK? When you think you are ready to try, come and see me.*

Scenario B:

- *What makes you consider to stop smoking? How interested are you in stopping smoking with my help? Can you grade to me from 1 to 10?*
- *How many years have you been smoking? How many cigarettes a day? Usually under what situations do you smoke?*
- *Have you tried to stop smoking before? What might be the reason of failure?*
- *Do you have any specific concerns? – Medical/social situation*

- *Well, This is an excellent decision you have made for your health. It may not be easy, especially at the beginning. You will experience withdrawal symptoms and urges. You may also feel stress, turn to eating and experience weight gain, etc.*

As your physician, I'll do everything I can to help you. Can you come back for another visit when we will have more time to talk about how we can do this together?

2nd visit

- *Review above, past attempts, compliance level*
- *Symptoms of withdrawal, address concerns*
- *Negotiate stop date, one day at a time*
- *Nicotine replacement therapy prescribed*
  Nicotine transdermal patch, nicotine-chewing pieces, explain use, and review chew technique
- *Behavior strategy*
  Avoid triggers: meals, coffee, alcohol, stress, routine
  Attitude-you are in control, rewards
  Stress management-relaxation, exercise, limit worrying
- *Offer ongoing help. If you need any help, please come and see me.*

29. Claudication

Case 1.

68 YOM with leg pain on walking, Do PE.
EKG: Left axis, left bundle branch block.
Risk factor: sedentary life style, smoking, high LDL.

Case 2.

52 YOM, claudication and calf pain for 6 months. History of varicose vein. PE
Interpret ECG, give risk factors, list investigations.

Keys:

Be aware of signs of critical ischemia:
  5Ps - pain, pulseless, parasthesia, pallor, paralysis
  Rest and night pain, ulceration, gangrene of toes, dependent
  rubor of soles and pallor on elevation.

PE

1. HEENT: look for xanthelasma indicate hypercholesterolemia
2. Pulse: rate, rhythm, contour, amplitude, ABI
3. Bruits: ausculate carotid, renal, abdominal aorta, iliac artery, femoral artery
4. BP supine/stand, both arm
5. JVP
6. Heart: murmur, signs of failure
7. Extremity:
 Inspect:
   Ulcer
   Skin color-pale or cyanosis
   Skin texture- atrophy
   Nail change– deformity
   Presence of hair-hair loss
   Muscle atrophy
   Edema or swelling
   Varicose veins

Palpate:
  Warm-temperature
  Pulse quality, localize site of blockage
  Tenderness along superficial vein
  Pitting edema
  Dependent rubor, pallor on elevation, elevation of leg, dangling
  on the side of Bed.

DDx

- *Arterial insufficiency:* presented with triad: calf discomfort on exertion, relieved by rest, reproducible pattern. PE reveals signs of chronic ischemia distal to obstruction.
- *Venous insufficiency:* Standing reveal dilated elongated superficial veins. Supine see discoloration of shins (hemosiderin deposit), pitting edema, painless ulcer located above medial malleolus. Trendeleburg test for vulvular competence.
- *Spinal stenosis/disk disease:* back pain, tenderness lateral to lumbosacral spine, ROM, sensory/motor/reflex exam of lower extremities, straight leg raise.
- *Other:* Cellulitis, DVT, phlegmasia alba dollen, phlegmasia cerula dollen

Interpret ECG, give risk factors, list investigations

- Look for left ventricular hypertrophy, old MI, and arrhythmia
- Risk factor: smoking, HTN, CAD, DM, hypercholestrol/-lipedemia
- Investigations: Ankle-brachial index (ABI), doppler U/S, arteriogram, venogram, treadmill testing, lumbar-sacral spine X-ray, CT, MRI, work up for risk factors

Chapter 2. Internal Medicine

1. Lymphadenopathy

Case 1.

Young female presents with night sweats and lymphadenopathy, which comes and goes. Obtain a focused history and perform a physical exam in 10 minutes. In the next 5 minutes, you are given a CXR that shows enlarged perihilar lymph nodes. List your differential diagnosis? What further tests would you order?

Key:

7 days $\Rightarrow$ Inflammatory; 7 months $\Rightarrow$ Tumor; 7 years $\Rightarrow$ Congenital

History:

General questions:

> *Age, occupation, past medical history, family history, medications, review of systems.*

Specific questions:

- *Onset: gradual/ sudden, progression, any other nodes?*
- *LN one side, both sides, distribution?*
- *Any fever, pain, and sore throat?*
- *Any Symptoms of erythema nodosum, watery/ red eye (uveitis), skin rash?*
- *Recent contact with ill persons? (Maybe her boyfriend has a sore throat) Mononucleosis: rash, spleen, and liver enlargement?*
- *Hx of drug use, STD, recent travel?*
- *Hx of URTI?*
- *Hx of exposure to TB, cough, hemoptysis?*
- *Evidence of non-palpable nodes:*
  Any Stridor / hoarseness-recurrent laryngeal?
  Any Cough dyspnea, facial swelling? (mediastinal nodes)
  Any Lower extremity edema? (retroperitoneal nodes)
- *Backache, urinary symptoms?*
- *Hx of malignancy: fatigue, weakness, wt loss, night sweats, abdominal pain, back pain, epigastric pain?*
- *Hx of anorexia, testicular mass, smoking, hemoptysis?*

Physical Exam:

- General appearance: Cachexia, anemia, fever, vitals.
- Head: occipital, posterior auricular or mastoid, parotid or preauricular lymph nodes.
- EENNT: Ear, eye, nose, nasopharynx, throat, oral cavity, Larynx, esp. large lymph nodes at upper neck.
- Thyroid.
- Virchow LN: left side GI, right side Lung, chest
- Examine cervical node, upper, lower, deep, superficial, anterior cervical chain
  Submaxillary, substyloid
- Abdomen: look for splenomegaly
- Look for other group of LN, name all the groups of LN you examined
- Liver, spleen.

Differential Diagnosis:

- Mononucleosis
- Metastatic tumor
- Drainage from an infection
- Sarcoidosis
- Lymphoma, Hodgkins/non-Hodgkins, Leukemia
- HIV
- Systemic lupus erythematous
- TB

Investigations:

- ACE level, non-specific for diagnosing sarcoidosis but it is good for signs of exacerbations.
- CXR, TB skin test (PPD), Acid-fast bacillus and sputum culture
- Complete blood count (CBC), blood smear, R/O hematologic disorders
- R/O metastasis from thyroid: U/S, CT, TSH, free T4, thyroid scan, FNA, biopsy.
- R/O metastasis from HENNT, GI and lung:
    Full otolargngologic exam
    Radiologic exam of GI, lung, sinus

- Pan-endoscopy include bronchoscopy, biopsy of normal tissue of nasopharynx, tonsils, base of tongue and hypopharynx.
- Excision, neck dissection

Case 2.

50 YOF presented with hilar adenopathy, list differential diagnosis and 6 blood tests indicating what to look for.

DDx (likely Dx in italics)

- Neoplastic - *Lymphoma,* bronchial carcinoma, metastatic tumors
- Inflammatory - *Sarcoidosis*
- Infectious - Tuberculosis, berylliosis, AIDS, etc

Blood tests

- CBC +Diff + peripheral blood smear - anemia of chronic disease, lymphopenia for HIV and sarcoidosis, increased immature lymphocytes for lymphoma
- Blood culture including acid fast bacilli
- Calcium, albumin, total protein-hypercalcemia in sarcoidosis, hyperglobulinemia in lymphoma and sarcoidosis.
- ACE level -elevated in sarcoidosis
- HIV serology if risk factors present

2. Hypothyroidism

Case 1.
40 YOF with hypothyroidism. Obtain a history.

Key:
Although 95% are due to primary causes. In this exam situation, you are likely to find a secondary cause.

History:
- *How do you feel?*
- *Any stiffness or cramping of muscles?*
- *Any numbness? Painful hand relieved by shaking/dangling/rubbing (Carpal tunnel syndrome)?*
- *Do you feel tired all the time?*
- *Any changes in your daily activity?*
- *Any problems with sleeping?*
- *Any change of appetite? Weight change?*
- *How frequent are you bowel movements?*
- *Any changes in your skin (dry), voice (hoarse), hair (dry), hearing loss (deafness may occur)?*
- *Have you noticed swelling in your legs? Face?*
- *Any changes in your menstrual periods?*
- *Do you like winter/summer? Do you need to wear more/fewer clothes than the rest of your family members?*
- *Any mood change (depression)? Ever thought about killing yourself? Vision/smell change?*
- *How long have you been like this? Is it getting worse/better? Can anything make it worse/better?*
- *Any other symptoms? Blurred vision, difficulty smelling?*

Etiology factors:
- *Ever noticed thyroid enlargement or puffy neck?*
- *Have you had neck surgery, thyroidectomy, pituitary surgery, or radiation therapy?*
- *Have you had an upper URTI recently with fever, sore throat and cough?*

- *Were you taking any anti-thyroid meds like lithium, iodine? Acetylsalicylic?*
- *Are there many people in your residential area that have the same problem?*
- *Ever felt neck pain, SOB?*
- *Are you pregnant?*

Differential Diagnosis:

<u>Primary:</u> 95%= Hashimoto's; postpartum; post-irradiation; subtotal thyroidectomy; Anti-thyroid drugs (lithium, PAS, PTU), Iodine deficiency, Biosynthetic defect; infiltrate (hemochromatosis, amyloidosis)

<u>Secondary:</u> Pituitary macroadenoma, empty sella syndrome, infarction, sarcoidosis, surgery, radiation

<u>Tertiary:</u> Hypothalamic induced.

3. Hypercalcimia

Case 1.
60 YOF found to have elevated serum calcium level x 2. Insurance company check up.

Case 2.
Hx. Bone pains over the hands, constipation, 2 important symptoms for DDx.

Case 3.
60 YOF Ca 3.0 and is asymptomatic, FHx of MEN, Focused Hx in 5 minutes.

Case 4.
50 year old female, hypercalcimia, Hx, PE, 3 likely diagnosis, 7 investigations and Management

Key:
MOANS, GROANS, STONES AND PSYCHOTIC OVER-
TONES for hyperparathyroidism/hypercalcemia

History:
General questions:
Age, occupation, past medical history, family history, medications, review of systems.

Specific questions:
- *Calcium level, how high? Repeat level the same? Interval of measurements?*
- *Any symptoms of*
        General: fatigue, weakness, weight loss, lethargy
        GI: constipation, pancreatitis, ulcer-PUD-stomach pain, anorexia, weight loss, constipation, nausea, vomiting, thirsty.
        CNS: confusion, psychosis, lassitude, depression
        GU: nephrolithiasis, renal insufficiency, urine frequency, polyuria, polydipsia

> *MS: myopathy, weakness, bone pain, arthralgia*
> *Other: HTN, metastatic calcification, band keratopathy*

- *Sx of underlying malignancy: cough, breast mass, bone pain, headache*
- *Intake of milk and antacids, thiazides, lithium, large dose of Vitamin D*
- *FHx of Hypercalcimia*

Differential Diagnosis:

- Hyperparathyroidism: primary, secondary, tertiary
- Malignancy: breast, lung (PTH like hormone), kidney, multiple myeloma
- Meds (thiazides or lithium)
- Immobilization
- Granulomatous disease (sarcoidosis)
- Familial hypocalciuric hypercalcemia
- Hyperthyroidism
- Addison's disease
- Excess ingestion of Vitamin D and Calcium
- MEN or hypocalciuric Hypercalcemia, milk alkali syndrome

Physical Exam:

- Vitals, commonly BP elevated, when dehydrated, orthostatic vital change
- MSE: confusion/encephlopathy
- Signs of malignancy: cachexia, Wt. Loss, breast mass, lung, abdx, LN, bone tenderness
- HEENT: parathyroid tumor, band keratinopathy, LN adnopathy (Sarcoidosis)
- MSK: bone/muscle weakness, hyporeflexia

Lab:

- PTH, PLP (PTH like protein), urine cAMP
- Basic metabolic panel(sodium, potassium, chloride, bicarbonate)
- PTH, $CaCl_2$ and PTH, ALP, Calcium Phosphate, X-ray subperiosteal bone absorption – hyperparathyroidism
- Anemia, ESR – multiple myeloma? – immunoelectrophoresis
- CXR hilar adenopathy +pulmonary finding + ACE – Sarcoidosis

- PLP, ALP, Bone Scan, spinal X-ray look for Metastasis
- Serum T3, T4 T3RU, TSH-r/o hyperthyroidism
- 24 hr Ca^{2+} excretion, serum vitamin D level

Case 4.

50 years old female, Hypercalcemia, Hx, PE, 3 likely diagnoses, 7 investigations and management.

Diagnoses:

1. Neoplastic disease – most common
- Tumors of lung, ovary, kidney – PLP; bone mets, multiple myeloma
2. Drug induced: thiazides, spirolactone, vitamine D intoxication
3. Milk-alkali syndrome

Others: MEN I/II, Zollinger-Ellison, hyper/hypo parathyroidism, adrenal insufficiency, sarcoidosis, immobilization

7 Investigations:

- Repeat Ca^{2+} level, with ionized Ca^{2+} level
- Serum/urine electrophoresis (SPEP, UPEP) CBC with differentiation (multiple myeloma)
- Lytes, BUN, Cr, ALP GGT
- 24 hr urine for Ca^{2+}, phos, Cr
- X-ray: chest, L/S spine, skull hands
- Other: PTH level, Urine cAMP

Management:

- IV fluids-NS 3-4L daily
- Ca^{2+} losing diuretic-lasix
- Diphosphonate
- Calcitonin
- ICU monitoring-cardiac
- Parathyroidectomy

4. Shock and Collapse

Case 1.
80 YOF, unconscious, in ER, HR 40/min, BP 80/40. Accompanied by granddaughter. Manage.

Case 2.
Collapsed in Mall, brought in by daughter. A-Fib Digoxin toxicity or low digestive level. hypovolemic due to diarrhea. Manage.

Assessment:
Primary Survey:
a. Turn on one side, clear airway, intubate

b. Oxygen 100% 5L/hr

c. Fluids, 2 Large IV, NS 1000 ml first hr, Cross match 10 units blood

d. Drug: give atropine, D/C digoxin, beta blocker, calcium channel blocker

e. Foley-urine output, ECG monitor, Vitals, Q15 min

Secondary Survey: Identify the cause

a. Hx from daughter:

• Activity at the time of fall, location, witness, trauma

• Symptoms before and after fall: dizziness, palpitation, dyspnea, chest pain, weakness, confusion.

* How quick to recover, pale or red during or after the attack

• Previous falls, AMPLE, previous CVD, CAD, Diabetes, seizure, HTN, Meds

b. Physical Exam:

Neurological: cerebellac-gait, Glascow coma scale, vision/hearing, Romberg test.

Cardiovascular: orthostatic BP change, arrhythmia, murmurs, carotid bruits

MSK: injury, joint, podiatric problems, ill fitting shoes

Abdomen: microcirculation.

Other: shoes, vision, hearing.

c. EKG 12 lead, Echo, CK-MB, angiogram, tropoman

d. CBC lytes, Glucose, PTT INR, Amylase BUN, Cr, ABGs

Definite treatment:

- Consult cardiology, external pacing may be required in the mean time
- Pacemaker, transcutaneous, transvenous
- PTCA, or by-pass surgery for MI

Case 3.

70 year old, collapsed in the mall, history and differential diagnosis

History:

- *Take history from a family member or observer whenever possible*
- *What were the exact circumstances of the black out?*
- *Did you have any warning of the attack?*
- *How quickly did you recover?*
- *Did you get pale or red during or after the attack?*
- *Are you taking any Meds?*
- *Shoes, vision, joint, hearing*

Differential Diagnosis:

- Epilepsy
- Vasovagal-micturition postural
- Vertebral basilar insufficiency
- Cardiac arrhythmia (block)
- Orthostatic hypotension

5. Hematuria

Case 1.
Old, male, find 50 RBC/HPF on routine urine analysis. Hx, Dx, 3DDx, 2 Investigations.

Key:
Make sure blood is from urine, not contaminated from stool or menstrual period.

History:
General questions:
Age, occupation, past medical history, family history, medications, review of systems.

Specific questions:
- *Gross or microscopic, painful or painless, with proteinuria or without?*
- *Any back or side pain and their onset, progression, radiation?*
- *Any change in the bowel movement? Any blood in stool?*
- *Female: menstrual Hx, make sure blood is from urinary tract and not vagina*
- *Which part of the urine is red: beginning, end or all the way through?*
- *How much blood? Any clots, what shape (worm shaped clot)*
- *Sx of urine frequency, dysuria, urgency, suprapubic pain, fever, STD?*
- *History of TB?*
- *Previous hx of kidney stone, Sx of renal colic*
- *Any difficulty in peeing? R/O BPH*
- *Any weight loss, night sweats? R/O tumor:*
- *Any changes in your diet or any medications worth mentioning? beets, dyes, rifampin?*
- *Have you been doing a lot of exercise recently, did you hurt yourself?*
- *Systemic-clotting problem, liver disease, taking anticoagulants, cancer treatment, analgesic use?*
- *FHx of polycystic disease, sickle cells disease?*

Physical Exam:
1. Presence of petechae, ecchymosis, lymphadenopathy, splenomegaly, anemia
2. Digital rectal exam (DRE): tender, bogy prostate
3. CVA tenderness or suprapubic tenderness
4. Bilaterally enlarged kidney-polycystic
   Unilaterally enlarged kidney-neoplasm or cyst
5. Presence of A-Fib or valvular heart disease suggests renal embolism or infarction
6. Signs of trauma

Differential Diagnosis:
　　　　Tumor　　Stone　　UTI　　BPH
Painless:
Age:　20-40 Calculus
　　　40-60 Renal Ca
　　　60-80 Bladder Ca, BPH
Painful:
- UTI, stone
- Acute hemmorrhagic cystitis, cyclophosphamide
Pseudo:
- Menses
- hemoglobinuria, myoglobinuria
- Dyes-beets
- Porphyuria
- Laxative-phsolaphalein
Less common:
- SLE, Sickle cell, GN, tense exercise

Investigations:
- Urine analysis, 3 glass test, IVP,
- Abdominal x-ray: Kidney ureter bladder (KUB), Flat plate and upright film
- Renal function, Cr-clearance, BUN, Cr, GFR
- U/S, CT, MRI
- Renal scan

- Cystoscopy, renal biopsy
- Immunologic studies: IgA, C3, C4
- Arteriography
- CBC-anemia, infection

Case 2.

56 YOM comes in for his annual check up. He has just returned from vacation. PE is normal. UA showed 50-100 RBC/HPF. He has lost some weight, no occult hematuria, has right costal vertebrae angle (CVA) pain, no other risk factors.

Q: List 3 DDx
   A: RCC, Stone, bladder Ca
Q: Investigations?
   A: Renal US, IVP, UA (casts, crystals, C+S, cytology), Cystoscopy

6. Renal Failure

Case 1.

48 YOF, Cr 1000. Obtain a history. What is your differential diagnosis and investigation?

Case 2.

Man with fatigue, Lab Cr 700. Obtain a history. What is your differential diagnosis? Investigate.

Case 3.

54 YOM presents with fatigue. He has a history of RF aggravated by captopril.

Key:

Don't miss the common things in the categorized differential diagnosis.

History:
Onset:

When were you aware of the elevation of Cr?
What happened at that time? Were you sick?
What do you mean by fatigue, do you have SOB when you walk?

Abrupt: *Did you have normal kidney function before?*

Chronic: *What kidney diseases have you had before? How is it being treated?*

- *Any problems with previous pregnancy?*
- *Do you notice any changes in sx?*
- *Aggravating/relieving factors?*

Pre-renal: *Allergy, medications, past medical history, last menstrual period, past examinations.(AMPLE).*

- *Do you have heart, liver, diabetes, HTN, serious illness/trauma/admission?*
- *Ever diagnosed with tumor? (tumor lysis), blood disease? Jaundice, (hemolysis), muscle trauma, muscle disease (rhibomyelysis)?*
- *Major surgery, hemmorrhage, hypertension?*

- *Any hypovolemia: GI loss, Skin loss, Renal loss, 3rd spacing?*

Renal:
- *Meds, NSAIDs, ACEIs radiography?*
- *Infection, fever, night sweats, urine burning, frequency?*
- *Any other skin hemorrhagic spots (petechiae=vasculitis)?*
- *Tumor, hematuria, weight loss*
- *Previous kidney disease*
- *FHx of polycystic renal disease*

Post renal:
- *Stone: abdominal pain?*
- *BPH: difficulty in passing urine (force, caliber, dripping)*
- *Incontinence: Are you able to control urination?*

Associated Sx:
- <u>*CNS*</u>*: confusion, inability to concentrate, fatigue, restless leg syndrome, neuropathy*
- <u>*CVS*</u>*: HTN, CHF, retinopathy*
- <u>*GI*</u>*: N/V, anorexia, UGI bleeding, constipation*
- *Skin rash, purpura, pigmentation*
- <u>*Endo*</u>*: hyperlipidemia, menstrual irregularity, low sex drive*
- <u>*Hemo*</u>*: anemia, bleeding, immune compromise*
- <u>*MSK*</u>*: nocturnal muscle cramping, joint effusion, leg edema*

Physical Exam: (Chronic Renal Failure)
- Sallow complexion, anemia – normocytic, normochromic
- bleeding, impaired cellular immunity – signs of infection
- pruritis, ecchymoses, hyperpigmentation
- Uremia fetor
- Deep acidic breathing (Kussmaul respiration)
- HTN
- Uremic encephlopathy-flapping tremor, mental clouding
- Pleural and pericardial effusion, pericardial rub (pericarditis)
- Evidence of fluid overload or depletion
- Renal mass (polycystic, etc)
- Large bladder-outlet obstruction

Investigation: 3 tests?
- Urine analysis, 24 hr urine, Cr clearance, blood BUN, Cr
- CBC, lytes, LFTs, BUN, Cr, ABG
- KUB x-ray
- IVP
- Renal scan
- U/s, CT, MRI
- Cystoscopy, renal biopsy

Differential Diagnosis:
Pre-renal:
- Volume depletion – hemorrhage, GI loss, third spacing, imadequate intake
- Reduce cardiac output - CHF, cardiogenic shock, tamponade
- Systemic vasodilation or vasoconstriction -spepsis, shock, drugs
- Systemic disease – Diabetes, HTN

Renal:
- Tubular ATN:
  Ischemia-hemorrhage, hypotension, surgery, burns
  Exo-toxin-radiocontrast, antibiotics
  Endotoxin. rhabomyolysis, hemolysis, tumor lysis
- Glomerular: recent infection
- Interstitium: acute interstitial nephritis (AIN), drugs, use of NSAIDs, ACEIs
- Vascular: malignant HTN, HUS/TTP
- Background kidney disease: chronic glomerular nephritis, polycystic kidney

Post renal:
- Ureter obstruction -blood clots, stones, tumors, papillary necrosis
- Urethra obstruction -stricture, prostate hypertrophy, tumor
- Infection

7. Diabetes

Case 1.
Diabetes counselling regarding diet/insulin/exercise.

Keys:
1. Get an idea of patient's condition first. Try to address patient's specific questions by asking "what questions do you have?" and start your consult from there.
2. Approach differently for type I and type II DM.

Questions you ask first:
a.   Onset, Sx, blood glucose level
* *Ask about excessive thirst?*
* *Ask about autonomic problems (impotence, incontinence, dizziness on standing, early satiety from gastroparesis.*
* *Ask about claudication (any pain in the back of legs when walking?)*
* *Ask about numbness and tingling of the feet?*
* *Ask about family history of diabetes?*

b. *Complications: heart, eye, renal, vascular, peripheral nerve, infection*
c. *Treatment: Diabeta, insulin, how much?*
d. *Weight: What do you eat each day? Weight change?*
e. *Ever loss of consciousness or seriously sick: DKA, hypo- hyperglycemia*
f. *Drugs, smoke, alcohol, other serious illness*
g. *Exercises: what, how much, how frequent, for how long?*

Diagnosis:
* Fasting plasma glucose>140mg/dl or 75g OGT 2hr/0-2hr >200mg/dl 7, 11
* Plasma glucose of>200 mg/dl in these patients is sufficient for diagnosis, no further testing is needed.

Consult – information you can provide:

Diagnosis and classification:

Diagnosis. Symptomatic patients will have polyuria, polydipsia, ketonuria and weight loss.

Type I: Insulin deficient, impaired secretion, Ketosis prone.

Type II. Obesity, insulin resistance

Complications: atherosclerosis, nephropathy, retinopathy, neuropathy, infection

Studies show: maintaining glucose level closer to normal can significantly reduce the risk of complications.

Diet:

a. Importance: Most type II DM can be controlled by achieving ideal body weight. The goal is gradual sustained weight reduction of approximately 1-2 lb/wk

b. Calculated nutrition +300-400 Kal for activity, -500 Kal for weight reduction lb/wk. Food 2/9 breakfast, 2/9 lunch, 4/9 dinner, 1/9 snack

c. Avoid simple sugars, saturated fat, excess salt. Take a high fiber diet, with complex carbohydrate and regular meals (50% carbohydrate 30%Fat 20%protein).

Exercise:

a. Benefit: Can deplete muscle glycogen, overcome insulin resistance

b. Insulin 1-2u per 20-30 min of activity, or take 15 gram carbohydrate, or change injection site to belly

c. Need stress test before rigorous exercise

d. Started with walking, 4-5 times per wk, 10-30 min, achieve 70-80% maxi-HR

Insulin:

a. Indication: all type I and decompensated type II

b. Store in fridge, draw accurately, inject site and rotation
Start dose 10-15 u, increase 1-2u/day until good control

Insulin starting at 0.5 U/kg with two thirds given in the morning

d. Divide dose: 2/3 Morning-1/3 regular, 2/3 intermediate
   1/3 Evening-1/2 regular before supper, ½ intermediate at bedtime

e. Continue insulin when you feel sick. May have insulin resistance when sick.

f. Signs of hypoglycemia: tremor, palpation, sweating-sympathomimetic and fatigue, confusion-neurologic

g. Have a syringe of glucogen ready

Monitor:
- Serum glucose, HB A1c, urine analysis, BUN, Cr; plasma lipids, ECG, ophthalmology annually

Case 2.
Dx DKA. Obtain a history, do a physical exam and manage.

Case 3.
52 YOM with diarrhea. Hx of DKA, manage.

Case 4.
IDDM clerk in a shop suddenly experiences an onset of severe headache and drowsiness. Do a physical exam and manage at ER. .

History:
- *When were you diagnosed with DM, How do you control your blood sugars?*
- *What is the cause of current situation? Infection, trauma, skip meds*
- *Now how do you feel? Headache, SOB, dizzy, N/V, confusion*
- *AMPLE*

Physical Exam:
- LOC, Vitals
- general appearance: Kussmaul breath, smell
- 'fruity' breath odor of acetone,

- Signs of dehydration (dry skin and mucous membranes and poor skin turgor), and altered consciousness to coma
- Signs of infection, trauma, etc
- Signs of insulin injection and DM complications
- Volume depletion

Investigation:

- CBC lytes glucose, ketone, ABGs, urine analysis, vitals EKG, ECG
- The diagnosis of DKA can be made by finding elevated blood glucose, increased serum levels of acetoacetate, acetone, and hydroxybutyrate metabolic acidosis (low serum bicarbonate and low blood PH), and increased anion gap.

Management:

- Rehydration 1L/hr NS for the first 2 hr, 2 large IV line
- Oxygen
- Insulin 10 u iv push, then 10 u/hr, hold s/c insulin for now
- Attention to K^+ with insulin
- Avoid bicarb

Other: if cerebral edema, mannitol

Manage in 1st hr:

- Volume: replace 3-5 L, NS 2000cc/1 hr, then 500cc/hr., then 150-200cc/hr
- Insulin: 5-10 U bolus then 50 u to 500 ml (0.1u/ml), 5-7u/hr
- K replacement when serum K level <4 meq/L
- What Lab parameters would you follow?: qhr glucose, K, lytes, urine output
- Monitor degree of ketosis with anion gap, not blood glucose or ketone level

8. Hypertension

Case 1.
19 YOF. BP 160/110. Hx, PE, 3DD, Investigation, Management.

Case 2.
50 year old university professor, BP 160/98, take a focus history. All tests and physical exam are normal, consult for treatment.

Keys:
- Confirm diagnosis
- R/o secondary cause
- R/o exogenous cause: alcohol, BCP, HRT-estrogen, NSAIDs
- Screen for target organ damage: angina/MI, TIA/stroke, claudication, RF (Cr>150)
- Screen for other cardiovascular risk factors: male, black, smoking, high cholesterol, DM
- Educate:

History:
- *Onset: When did you notice your BP was high? When was your last normal BP?*
  Ask about diet? exercise?
  Ask about stresses in life, employment or family?
  Ask if cholesterol level is known?
- *Changes: How high was it? Were you treated? How high is it now?*
- *Complications: Have you had chest pain, SOB, claudication, vision change, stroke?*
- *Suggest secondary:*
  Notice any change in your body? Voice, hair, bruising?
  Do you have episodes of sweating, palpation, headache?
  Are you taking any medications? Amphetamine, birth control pill (BCP), licorice, thyroid hormoe?
  Do you have diabetes or kidney disease?
- *PMHx: Do you smoke, drink, or use drugs?*
- *SHx: Do you like salty diet? Any weight gain recently?*

- *FHx: Any family member with high BP?*

Physical Exam:
1. Diagnosis and severity
- Recheck BP, Measure BP on both sides, arms and legs.
- Check the blood pressure when sitting and standing.
- Feel at least 2 pulses: carotid, radial, posterior tibialis, etc.
2. Possible cause
- Signs of coarction of aorta: simultaneous radial/femoral pulse palpation
- Signs of pheochromacytoma: pallor, tachycardia, sweating, headache
- Signs of Cushings: striae, pigmentation, central obesity
- Signs of Renal disease: edema (renal)
- Renal bruits, big kidney (polycystic)
- Signs of neurofibromatosis, thyroid, muscle tone, proximal myopathy.
3. End organ damage
- Examine fundi
- Examine heart and lungs, heart murmur, pulmonary edema
- Carotid pulse/bruits, neurology sign
- Peripheral vascular pulse bruits, capillary refill
- Abdomen mass and bruits

Differential Diagnosis and Investigation:
- Estrogen: approximately 5% taking BCP will exhibit a rise in BP above 140/90, less common in those taking low dose estrogen tablets.
- Renal: nephritic/nephrotic syndrome,
- Renal vascular: young-fibromuscular dysplasia, older-atherosclerotic disease
- Adrenal: Cushings, Primary aldosteronism (hypokalemia), pheochromacytoma
- Cushings, – Pheochromacytoma, – Coarction of aorta
- Hyperthyroidism
- HTN associated with pregnancy

- Patients <25 or>45 years old with new hypertension should be examined closely for secondary causes of hypertension.

DD	Screen	Confirm
Coarction of aorta	CXR	angiography
Cushings	1mg Dexamethasone (-) test	High dose (-) test
Pheochromacytoma	24 hr urine VMA, metanephrine	Angiography, CT
Renal	urine analysis, BUN Cr	Cr clearance, IVP, U/S, Biopsy
Renal vascular	Captopril renal scan	Angiography Differential renal vein rennin

IF all results normal, initiate management.

1 Smoking cessation
2 Salt and alcohol restriction
3 Weight reduction if >115% of ideal body weight
4 Regular aerobic exercise
5 Behavior therapy: modify environment/events to reduce stress
6. All these for 3-6 months no response then Pharmacological: low dose thiazide diuretic <50 mg/day

9. Anemia

Case 1.

Young lady comes for PE in order to enroll with the RCMP. (a) Take a relevant history. HB and reticular count abnormal. (b) What other blood test would you do (TIBC, iron, VitB12, foliate). What are 3 things from the history that lead to a diagnosis (heavy period, poor diet, etc); advise about diet.

Key

Bleeding; Inadequate production; Excessive destruction

History:

* *When started, any changes over time?*
* *Notice any bleeding GI GU? How about your period?*
* *What is your diet like?*
* *Giadiasis: How frequent are BMs? What is the stool like? Any cramping?*
* *Malignancy: Any fever, night sweats, adenopathy or wt change?*
* *Any chronic disease, liver, kidney?*
* *Genetic: What is your ethnic background (Mediterranean)? Any family members anemic?*
* *Hemolysis: Do you feel itchy (jaundice)? What does your urine look like?*
* *B12 deficiency:*
  Hx of gastric surgery, inflammatory bowel disease, hypothyroidism, raw fish intak?
  Any Vitiligo, glossitis and neuropsychiatric Sx?
* *Foliate deficiency:*
  Hx of alcohols, poor nutrition, pregnancy, blood dyscrasia, spruce, psoriasis, anti-convulsant, anti-metabolite therapy?

Case 2.

69 YOM, fatigue, dizziness, unsteady gait for a few weeks. Lab. MCV 120, HB 90, WBC 3.4, Hx, Dx, 2 Investigations.

History:

He has diarrhea, sensory ataxia,: ETOH abuse
Megablastic anemia
Q: What supports your DX?
Sensory ataxia, high MCV, low HB
Q: What do you call this neurological syndrome?
Combined degeneration of the spinal cord
Q: Investigations?
Shillings test, Bone marrow analysis
B12 level, blood smear

10. Angina, Acute Myocardial Infarction

Case 1.

55 YOM with 1 hour history of crushing retrosternal chest pain, BP 110/80, HR 180, irregular. Take a focused history and perform a physical exam in 10 minutes.

Case 2.

Chest pain: interpret ECG changes-Ischemia+MI

Case 3.

Diagnosis is an acute MI. Obtain a history and perform a physical exam in 10 minutes. List a management plan in the next 5 minutes.

Case 4.

80 YOM presents with chest pain, SOB, and history of IHD. Perform a physical exam, CXR and ECG.

Key:

- Be sympathetic; always address patient's anxiety, worries and concerns.
- OLDCARS (Onset, Location, Duration, Character, Associate Sx, Radiation, Severity.
  OPQRST: (Onset, Precipitating, Quantity, Relieving, Severity, Timing.)

History:

- *Do you get pain in your chest on exertion, e.g. climbing stairs? Have you experienced symptoms at rest?*
- *How many blocks you can walk without symptoms appearing (chest pain)?*
- *Where is the pain located?*
- *Does it radiate to other places?*
- *Is it getting worse on cold air or exercise after a big meal?*
- *Is it bad enough to stop you from exercising?*
- *Does it go away when you rest? How long does it take?*
- *Do you ever get similar pain if you get excited or upset?*

- *Onset:*

  When? Any similar pain before? Suddenly or gradually?

  What happened at home, work? Any stress? Strain muscles, cough?
- *Location: Can you point to the place that hurts the most?*
- *Duration: How long usually the pain will last? Minutes, hours.*

  Any changes in duration recently?
- *Character:*

  Can you describe your pain for me? What is it like? Heaviness, cutting, ache, burning?

  What situation would likely cause the pain? Eating, exercise, coughing.

  Can you relieve the pain by rest, sitting and leaning forward (pericarditis), or taking nitroglycerin?
- *Associated symptoms:*

  Do you have SOB, N/V, fever, weight loss?

  How frequent are you having the pain? Any changes in frequency of the pain, recently?

  Do you have heartburn, acid reflux and dysphasia?

  Have you seen any Dr before? What tests have been done? What Meds were given?

  Have you ever used streptokinase? Allergy

  How severe, can you grade it from 1 to 10?
- *Radiation:*

  Does the pain stay in the chest or does it radiate to the arm, back, shoulder?
- *PMH:*

  AMPLE (Allergy, Medications, Ptk, Last menstrual period, Events)

  Do you have diabetes, HTN, gastric- esophageal disease?

  Do you drink, smoke, using drugs, taking Meds?

  Have you ever had surgery, immobilization, trauma, leg swelling, taking heparin, BCP, pregnancy, pleuritic chest pain, chronic venous insufficiency, inactivity?

Physical Exam:
Keys:

1. Place patient in a comfortable position: Sitting up – pulmonary edema, Lie down – hypovolemic or PE

2. While taking history, watch for easily visible signs such as hand warmth, sweating, peripheral cyanosis, clubbing, nail splinter hemorrhage, JVP.

Closer look:
Face, conjunctiva, tongue, inside the mouth

BP:

- Both arms, supine and upright
- Orthostatic hypotension: SBP drop >20, DBP drop >10
- Pulse pressure
- Pulse alterans
- Pulse paradoxus-drop >10 during inspiration

Arterial pulse:
- Rate, rhythm, amplitude, contour

Auscultate for bruits:
- In carotid, AA, temporal, renal, iliac and femoral A
- JVP

Expose chest
- Inspection: Precardial apex beat, heaves, lifts, location, size, quality, thrils, breathing pattern, any abnormal pulsation
- Palpation: Palpate precordium, locate the apex beat and assess its character. Any abnormal vibrations or thrills
- Pulmonary auscultation: Both front and back for pleural effusion (heart border), cracks at lung base.
- Heart auscultation: Heart sounds/murmur; timing, duration, rate, rhythm, pitch, intensity, pattern, quality, location, radiation, relation to respiration, .splitting, extra sounds, opening snap, clicks, and pericardial rubs, carotid artery-radiating murmur or bruits,

Abdomen:
- Lie flat, palpate liver, Aortic Aneurysm.

Leg:
- Check femoral, popliteal, dorsalis pedis and posterior tibialis pulses.
- Look for ankle or sacral edema

If appropriate, assess the patient's exercise tolerance with a walk.

- **ECG basics:**
- Rate
- Rhythm: P waves present? QRS wide or narrow? P and QRS relation? Regular rhythm or not?
- Axis: normal positive QRS on I an II
- Waves and segments
- Hypertrophy and chamber enlargement
- Ischemia and infarction
- Miscellaneous: Hyper/hypo- Kalemia, Calcemia

Management of the MI patient:
1. ABCs-stabilize
2. 12-lead EKG; cardiac monitor,
3. Previous EKG to compare?
4. Oxygen by mask
5. Sublingual nitroglycerin x3 r/o angina
6. Morphine 2mg IV
7. Aspirin 325 mg chew stat
8. Beta Blocker, lasix if BP OK, if BP low, consider PTCA/ emergent bypass
9. Thrombolysis: r-tPA start within 6hrs of onset
10. CXR and blood work: CBC, cardiac enzyme, amylase, ABG

Then consider:
1. ACE inhibitors
2. Heparin
3. Coumadin x 3months
4. Lipid-lower agents
5. Nitrates

11. Pneumonia, Pleurisy

Case 1.
30 YOM c/o: right-side chest pain. Pain more severe with deep breathing, no SOB. Perform a physical exam.

Case 2.
25 YOM with fever and pleuritic chest pain. a) perform a physical exam, b) read CXR, c) what is your treatment?

Case 3.
27 YOM presents with chest pain, fever, cough. High WBC, high temperature.

Case 4.
Approach a patient with pneumonia who is an alcoholic and smoker. Obtain a history and consult.

Case 5.
Patient with pneumonia/cough. Perform a physical exam, X-ray and manage.

Key:
Distinguish bacterial from non-bacterial etiology is critical for treatment.

History:
OLDCARS
Have you had any of:
- *Dyspnea: PND/orthopnea, episodic SOB, exercise tolerance, life style-activity?*
- *Cough: productive, wheezy, nocturnal, positional cough, change in cough pattern?*
- *Sputum: color, blood, purulent, green, frothy pink, red current jelly?*
- *Fever, have you taken your temperature? How high?*
- *Chest pain? Association with breathing-pleurisy?*
- *Do you drink? Were you drunk the day before? How drunk, ever lost*

conscious? Similar episode before? Head trauma, intoxication, neurological disorder? – aspiration.

- *Other associated sx: diarrhea, confusion, bradycardia – legionella pneumonia*
- *PMHx, allergy, eczema, TB, respiratory infection, chronic lung disease? History of HIV, PCP, CMV, mycobacterium infection? Recent URTI?*
- *SHx, occupation, smoking, pets, recent travel?*
- *Family History: asthma, eczema, allergies, TB contact.*

PE:
Respiratory System
- Vitals
  While taking history, and talking with patient, watch for respiratory distress and clues from the surrounding, nasal flare, pursed lip breathing, using of accessory muscles, indraw.
- Posture: sitting upright, use pillows
- Clubbing, cyanosis (central, peripheral) nicotine stain
- CO_2 retention: tremor, headache, and warm periphery, pounding pulse
- JVP-cor pulmonae, CHF
- Supra-clavicular LN
- Chest:

Inspection:
- Pattern of breathing, rate, rhythm, depth
- Chest wall deformity and inequality: Barrel chest, kyphosis, scoliosis, pectus excavatum, flail chest, retractions, and contractions

Palpation:
- Displacement of trachea; chest wall tenderness, vocal fremitus; crepitus, pericardial pulsation; chest expansion

Percussion:
- In sequence, dullness, hyper resonance, diaphragmatic excursion

Auscultation:
- Overt adventitious sounds – wheeze, noise vocal resonance, whisper pectoriloquy, added sounds, decreased breath sounds, wheezes, pleural friction rub, adventitious sound, transmitted sound
- ·If appropriate, measure flow rate

Heart: auscultation... S3 gallop (CHF)

X-Ray: PA and lateral
- Patchy and diffuse infiltrate:
  Atypical-legionella, mycoplasma, viral, aspiration, PCP
- Segmental or lobar:
  Pnemococcal infection.
- Parapneumonic effusion:
  Complications-abscess, emphysema, pneumathorax

Consult:
a. Good fluid intake
b. Temperature taken every evening
c. Avoid overuse of cough suppression. Use only at night for sleep. Cough helps to clear the airway
d. Cease smoking
e. Watch for evidence of worsening: unremitting fever, drowsiness, dyspnea, and cyanosis.

Emergency Room Treatment:
Community acquired typical Pneumonia:
- Penicillin 2 million units IV q4h and cefuroxime 750mg IV q8h

Community acquired atypical Pneumonia:
- Erythromycin 500 mg IV qid and to PO ASAP
- 1g IV q6h for legionella

Aspiration Pneumonia:
- Penicillin 2 million units IV q4h or Ampicillin 1g IV q6h or
- Clindamycin 600mg IV q6h for bacteroides plus gentamycin 1.5 mg/kg IV q8h or
- Ceftazidine 1g IV q8h

Nursing home or nosocomial Pneumonia:
- Cefuroxime 750mg tid + gentamycin, or
- Ceftriaxone 1g IV/IM q12h, or
- Pipercillin 2g IV q4h +tobramycin for high risk pseudomonas infection

If at risk of aspiration:

- Clindamycin 600mg q8h +gentamycin 1g q8h, or
- Flagyl 500 mg tid + cefotaxime 1-2g q8h, or
- Imipenem 500 mg IV q6h

Pneumococcal infections: penicillin;
H. influenza: Ampicillin or amoxicillin;
Mycoplasmal/Q-fever/psittacoses: tetracycline;
Legionnaires` disease/Morexella: erythromycin

12. Chest Pain, Physical Exam.

Case 1.
38 YOM with sudden onset of chest pain and cough. Perform a physical exam. CXR: pneumathorax.

Case 2.
65 YOM had THR and is presently admitted to the floor because of dyspnea and chest pain. Perform physical exam. PE, vs fat emboli.

Key:
• Examine chest wall, heart, lung, be gentle.
• Comment on why and how you do the exam.

PE:
* General appearance: level of consciousness, vitals, CVS, JVP cyanosis, breath pattern (anxiety)--rate, rhythm
• Skin: Herpetic rash, pallor, jaundice, xanthomata, anemia, SO2
• Carotid pulse, bruits
• Chest: As in Case 2
• Abdomen:
  Palpation for: tenderness, mass especially AAA, liver, spleen
  Auscultation for: bowel sounds and bruit
• Legs:
  Edema, phlebitis, vascular insufficiency, signs of DVT, measure calf circumference in both sides, peripheral pulsus.
• Cervical and Thoracic spine and neurology sign.

DDx:
• Chest wall: Muscle spasm, strain, Tietze's, rib fracture, cervical/thoracic spine-nerve root compression, herpes, Ca invasion, Mets
• Cardiac: Ischemic, pericarditis
• Lung and pleural: Pneumothorax, PE, pneumonia, bronchospasm
• GI, GE: Reflux, spasm, ulcer, cholecyctitis, pancreatitis
• Psychogenic: Anxiety, depression, malingering

• Fat emboli

Investigations:

• ECG, CXR, V/Q scan, and cardiac enzymes, ABGs

13. Pulmonary Embolism, Anticoagulant Use, Consult.

Case 1.
60 YOF. History of pulmonary embolism, doesn't take Coumadin after discharge from hospital. Consult.

Case 2.
60 YOF diagnosed with pulmonary embolism is hospitalized. On Coumadin PT 17, control 11. INR correction factor-PT=11 control 11. What would you tell the patient? Obtain a history and provide counselling.

Consult:
- Ask when and why this meds was prescribed, *Why you are not taking meds? Any particular side effects you are concerned about?* How much the patient already knows:
- *Anticoagulants have been prescribed for your current medical problem (PE, MI). It decreases the clotting ability of the blood and therefore prevents harmful clots from forming in the blood vessels. These meds are sometimes called blood thinners, although they don't actually thin the blood. They do not dissolve clots that already have formed, but they prevent clots becoming larger and causing more serious problems.*
- *If you are allergic to any anticoagulants or any food products (like sulfates or other preservatives) or if you are on a special diet (like low salt, low sugar), please let me know.*
- *We recommend normal, balanced diet.*
- *If you begin using any new meds or if you develop any new medical problem while you are using this Meds, please let me know*
- *Anticoagulants may cause birth defects. Don't take this med during pregnancy and don't become pregnant while taking this med.*
- *This medicine is especially sensitive in very young or very old with increased chance of bleeding.*
- *Make sure you don't have any of the following conditions or medical procedures:*
    Childbirth
    Fall or blows to the body or head

Fever lasting for more than a couple of days
Heavy or unusual menstrual bleeding
Insertion of IUD
Medical or dental surgery
Severe or continuing diarrhea
Spinal anesthesia
X-ray (radiation) treatment

- *Take this med only as directed. If you miss a dose, take it as soon as possible. If you don't remember until the second day, don't take the missed dose. Doubling dose may cause bleeding.*
- *I will check your blood daily x5days, then every 3 days x2weeks, then weekly*
- *Tell all medical doctors, dentists and pharmacists you go to that you are taking this Med. Or carry a Med ID stating that you are using this meds*
- *Avoid any injuries (sports, cutting). If happened, report to doctor earlier as serious internal bleeding may occur*
- *Storage:*
  a. out of reach of children
  b. away from heat or direct light or moisture; discard outdated meds
- *After you stop taking this med. (usually 6 months), it takes time for your blood clotting ability to return to normal. Use caution.*
- *Any questions?*

14. Paroxysmal Atrial Tachycardia, Atrial Fibrillation, On Digoxin, Consult

Case 1.
60 YOF complains of paroxysmal atrial tachycardia; she is on digoxin. Pulse irregular on exam. Explain the need for meds to the patient.

Case 2.
60 YOF. Previously admitted in CHF, secondary to A-fib, returns for check up. Digoxin level is sub therapeutic. Consult her regarding her illness and her Meds.

Focus History :
* *When were you diagnosed A-Fib (or PAT)? What is your symptom at that time?*
* *Is the heart beat regular or irregular? Could you tap on the table the rate you think your heart goes during an attack?*
* *Anything set attacks off? Does it happen at rest? During activity? After a meal? Are there any foods that seem to make the symptom worse?*
* *How frequent does it happen? How long does it normally last?*
* *Can you do anything to stop the attack? What did you do when you had an attack?*
* *What meds are you taking? When you started taking Digoxin? Does digoxin make you feel better?*
* *How much is the dose prescribed? How much are you actually taking now?*
* *Is there a special reason that makes you decide to take less meds?*
* *What Symptoms do you have now? SOB, palpation, fatigue, leg swelling? Does the Symptom get worse when you exercise?*
* *Can I feel your pulse?*
* *Do you drink, smoke, use any other Meds?*
* *AMPLE diabetes, HTN, hyperlipidemia, FHx*
* *Now can you tell me what you know about A-Fib (or PAT) and how digoxin works?*
* *Any particular concerns or fears about this treatment?*

Consult:

- Check on compliance and realize that the reason for noncompliance is because she is concerned about the side effects of digoxin. She asks about: the need of these Meds, duration of therapy, side effects, F/U and how often, when to omit the dose. What will happen when she goes to Florida on a holiday, etc?

- Reassure her that it is necessary to control her heart rate, and there is minimum toxicity if in the therapeutic range. Take the usual dose. Arrange to recheck digoxin level after 1 week. Ask her to let you know if she was put on any other medications, so that you can monitor drug interactions e.g. Cimetidine, Theophyline, Phenobarbital, etc. Tell her about the side effects to watch for: blurred or yellow vision, headache, drowsy, green color blindness, nausea, syncope, etc

- Our heart is like a pump. Your heart problem is it beats too fast and irregular. If it can't effectively pump blood to your system, you'll have symptoms of heart failure including c/p, SOB, headache ... It can also cause stroke, peripheral thromboembolism because blood clot will easily form when you hear beating like that.

- Digoxin will slow your heart down and makes it beat stronger. On a therapeutic dose, the side effects are minimal. The side effects to watch for: blurred or yellow vision, headache, drowsy, green color blindness, nausea, syncope, etc
- Your problem is that you are not getting enough digoxin in your system. I am going to ask you to take the prescribed dose and ask you to come back in a weeks time to see how you are doing and to check your drug level. Is that all right with you? After that I'll have a better feeling about what dose should be taken when you are on vacation in Florida. However, anytime if you have any symptoms mentioned above, or you starting any new meds or simply you are concerned about anything, feel free to call or come to see me, OK? Any questions?

15. Hemoptysis– Cardiac Failure

Case 1.
60 YOM complains of scant hemoptysis, and short of breath (SOB).
a) Take a history, Dx, DDx.
b) CXR, ECG indicate MI, LVF, manage.

Key:
Assess severity and find etiology.

History:
General questions:
Age, occupation, past medical history, family history, medications, review of
  systems.
  AMPLE
Specific questions: OLDCARS
For Breathlessness
* *Does SOB happen on exertion?*
* *How much can you do before getting SOB?*
* *Do you ever wake up at night gasping for breath?*
* *If so, do you have to sit up or get out of bed?*
* *How many pillows do you sleep on?*
* *Do you cough or wheeze when you are are having SOB?*
* *Is the SOB at activity, rest or PND?*

For Hemoptysis
* *How are you feeling now? Do you feel dizzy? Headache?*
  hemodynamically stable?
* *Are you coughing up blood or vomiting blood?*
* *Do you have a nose bleed? Teeth bleed?*
* *Is this something new or does it happen every spring/winter (COPD,*
  brochiolitis)?
* *When did it start? Suddenly or gradually?*
* *What does the sputum look like?*
* *Gross bloody or pink (LVF) or putrid (lung abscess) or copious amount of*
  purulent sputum mixed with blood (bronchioectasis)?
* *Any chest pain, fever? How high is the temperature? – pneumonia, MI*

- *Any night sweats or weight loss? -Cancer*
- *Do you smoke? How much a day? How many years? – Cancer*
- *Have you had TB before or recent contact with TB?*
- *Previous bleeding somewhere else? – gum bleed, skin bruising?*
- *How is your urine output? Any problems with your kidney function?*
- *Ever notice blood in the urine? (Goodpasture`s disease)*
- *Have you recently had surgery or long-distance air travel?(PE)*
- *Any family member having similar problems? Pulmonary AVM i.e. Osler-weber-rendu*
- *Did you catch a cold?*
- *Are you on any Meds-anticoagulants?*

Manage:

In sequence:
1. Treat underlying disease: CAD, HTN, hyperthyroidism, hypothyroidism
2. Treat precipitating factors: anemia, fever, pneumonia, PE, exertion, emotion, and high dose beta-blocker
3. Salt restricted diet (2 gr daily)
4. Diuretics (can't use in AS)
5. ACE inhibitor: Captopril
6. Digoxin need monitor HR, rhythm, serum K, Mg
7. Other: anticoagulation, avoid calcium channel blockers, beta-blockers
- If arrhythmia present, amiodarone is first choice.

Differential Diagnosis (in Hemoptysis and SOB):

Heart: • Congestive heart failure
- Fatigue, syncope, hypotension, cool extremity

Lung: • Bronchioectasis, endotracheal malignancy, PE, pneumonia
- Chronic cough, recurrent respiratory infection, occupation exposure, heavy smoking
- Pulmonary AVM in Osler-weber-rendu, family history

Psycho: Multiple body complaints, history of emotional difficulties, lack of activity, exacerbation, chest tightness, suffocation, or inability to take in air

16. Lung Nodule, Cancinoma, Tuberculosis

Case 1.
Female patient found to have a nodule on routine CXR. Perform a focused physical exam. What is your differential diagnosis?

PE
Inspection:
a. Skin: teleangiectasia, cyanosis (central, peripheral), nicotine stain, cachexia, jaundice.
b. Distress: nasal flare, pursed lip breathing, accessory muscle use
c. Posture: sitting upright, use of pillows
d. Chest shape: horizontal-emphysema, barrel – COPD, Kyphosis/scoliosis, pectus excavatum, flail
Palpation:
a. LN: at sub- super- clavicular and axillary area
b. Mass and tenderness
c. Tactile fremitus
d. Trachea, breath excursion
Percussion:
a. Dull/Tympanic
b. Diaphragmatic excursion
Auscultation:
a. A/E, wheeze
b. Friction rub
c. Audible bruit

Investigation:
- CXR
- CT, MRI
- Sputum cytology
- Bronchoscopy
- Mediastinoscopy
- FNA
- VATS and throcotomy

Differential Diagnosis:

Infectious:

• Healed granuloma: tuberculous, histoplasmosis, coccidiomycosis

Neoplasm:

• Benign: Harmatoma
• Malignant: Primary or metastatic: from breast, colon, testicles, etc

Congenital:

• Bronchogenic cyst, hydatid cyst, pseudo lymphoma, A/V malformation, bronchopulmonary sequestration

Extra pulmonary:

• Skin, nipple, chest wall, rib, pleural plaque

Favor carcinoma:
    Speculated, irregular or lobulated edge
    Presence of other coin lesions
    Associated mediastinal adenopathy or boney metastasis
    Growth compared to an earlier film
    Obstructive phenomenon-peripheral consolidation/atelectasis.
Unlikely carcinoma:
    Calcification
    Cavity with darker center compared to the circumference
    Air fluid level suggest abscess

Case 2.

50 year old male smoker and current textile worker has a likely diagnosis of lung cancer. Consult.

Consult:

• *How much do you know already?*
• *What more would you like to know about your disease?*
• *What is on your mind?*
• *Provide clear diagnosis and staging, possible cause, explain Symptoms.*
• *There are major differences in prognosis based on tissue type and staging, prognosis for this particular patient needs to be explained.*

- Treatment options:

Non-small cell: Stage I/II– surgery; Stage III-palliative

Small cell: Local-surgery after radiation; Extensive-chemo, radiation

- Provide information, form a joint plan, respect patients wishes.
- Facilitating communication between family and patient

Case 3.

Female immigrant, abnormal CXR screening for work. History of exposure to TB. She has experienced weight loss and night sweats, but no cough. Obtain a history. CXR compatible to TB, what are other possible differential diagnoses?

History:

- *When did you take this X-ray? When was the last time you had a CXR? The newly discovered abnormality is?*
- *How old are you? When did you start smoking? How much do you smoke?*
- *Do you cough? What is the sputum looks like? Any blood in the sputum?*
- *Any hx of previous malignancy? testicle, breast, colon Ca,?*
- *Do you have bone pain, headache, and weight loss? How much weight loss in what time period?*
- *Exposure to TB: Any family or friends have TB?*
- *What job do you have? Do you have any contact with bird feces? histoplasmosis, Coccidiomycosis*

X-ray: heavy calcified old granuloma

DDx: Mycobacterium Avium, HIV, lymphoma, Lung primary/Metastatic Ca, Atypical pneumonia or fungal infection.

17. Asthma

Case 1.
Patient with cough for 2 wks, asthmatic, green sputum, on ß-blocker + ventolin. Obtain a history in 5 minutes.

Key:
Try to identify triggering factor.

History:
General questions:

Age, occupation, past medical history, family history, medications, review of systems.

Specific questions:
- *When were you diagnosed with asthma?*
- *What triggers an attack? Exercise, cold, pets, etc?*
- *Do you have chronic symptoms? Are you on regular meds?*
- *Are you a cougher or a wheezer?*
- *Do your symptoms get worse at night?*
- *Are you allergic to anything?*
- *Anybody smoke at home? Any pets?*
- *Any family members with asthma?*
- *When were you started on beta blocker? Did your symptoms get worse after that?*

18. Aortic Stenosis

Case 1.

60 YOM, asymptomatic, with a heart murmur found by family doctor. Perform a physical exam. Ejection systolic murmur at left sternum border and radiate to the carotids: Diagnosis is: Aortic Stenosis. Consult.

Physical Exam:

- Carotid pulse: slow upstroke and late peaking, thrill over carotid and suprasternal notch
- Sustained precordial palpation, systolic thrill at 2nd right intercostals space (RICS)
- Systolic ejection murmur (SEM), diamond shaped, radiate to neck with paradoxical splitting of S2

Consult:

Asymptomatic patients:

- have excellent survival (near normal)
- Close F/U for symptoms and with serial echocardiograms.
- Supportive/medical: avoid heavy exertion; infectious endocarditis prophylacsis; avoid nitrates/vasodilators; treat CHF

Symptomatic patients:

- Need surgery because if untreated has high mortality: usually die within 5 yr after onset of syncope, 3 yr after onset of angina and <2yr after onset of CHF/dyspnea
- It is the most fatal valvular lesion. Cause of death – V-Fib, left ventricular failure, complete heart block.

19. Upper GI Bleeding, Management

Case 1.
60 YOF, presented with hematemesis, Manage

Case 2.
30 YOM, hemoptysis, abdominal pain. In apparent distress in emergency department. BP 80/50. Give orders to nurse.

Keys:
Make sure bleeding is from GI source
Following sequence: ABC, stabilize, focused Hx and PE, then definitive treatment

Stabilize the patient:
- ABCs. Ask if the patient is in a coma or awake, if in coma, intubate.
- Two large bore IV, ensure hemodynamic stability, give crystalloid/plasma/blood as needed.
- NG tube: to see if the bleeding is from upper GI source, empty stomach if it is. Balloon tamponade
- Initial Lab test: type and screen, cross match 6-10 units of blood. CBC HB, PTT/INR.
- Other: ECG monitor, oxygen, elevate foot end of the bed. Monitor urine output.

Hx:
- *How much did you vomit? Is the blood coughed up?*
  Hematemesis usually indicates bleeding site proximal to Treitz ligament.
- *What does the vomitus look like? What color? Any clots?*
  It is associated with speed of bleeding, also indicate continuous bleeding if vomit red fresh blood. If blood stays in the stomach for a while, it will look like coffee grounds.
- *Have you had BM? What is the stool like?*

Bleeding sufficient to produce hematemesis usually results in melana as well, whereas less than half of patients with melana have hematemesis.

- *Any symptoms of syncope, light headness, sweating, thirst, angina?*
  Indications of large volume blood loss.
- *Have you feel discomfort with you stomach recently? Previous surgery or treatment for ulcer?*
  Symptoms of epigastric pain, sharp/burning/gnawing, relief with food/antacids indicate peptic ulcer disease.
- *Any history of alcohol use or liver disease?* Indicate varices bleeding
- *What meds are you taking?*
  History of anti-inflammatory medications – NSAIDS
- *Were you vomiting before blood appears?*
  History of retching prior to hematemesis – Mallory-Weiss
- *Lost any weight recently?*
  History of weight loss – Carcinoma

PE:

- Vital signs: tachycardia, orthostatic hypotension, pallor, diaphoresis, cool skin, JVP
- Oral/nasopharynx to exclude non-intestinal bleeding source
- Stigmata of chronic liver disease: spider angioma, gynecomastia, testicular atrophy, jaundice, ascites, hepatosplenomegaly
- Abdomen for tenderness, mass lesion, etc
- Rectal exam, color of stool

Then:
Consult gastroenterologist for endoscopy and definitive treatment
1. Peptic ulcer disease: cauterize visible vessels, inject epinephrine, triple therapy for H Pylori-clarithromycin, metronidazole, proton-pump inhibitor
2. Gastritis: treat H pylori or other offending agents – alcohol, NSAIDS, etc
3. Varices: banding, sclerosing, portal-systemic venous shunt (TIPSS), beta-blockers, Sigura procedure – surgical esophageal transection, etc.
4. Mallory-Weiss. Consult general surgery if necessary

20. Acidemia

Case.
55 YOF with arterial blood gas show acidemia, assess.

A: Check PH: Acidemia or Alkalemia?
B: Differentiate respiratory versus metabolic
  – Respiratory:
  PCO_2 opposite to pH
  PCO_2 high, HCO_3 high
  – Metabolic:
  HCO_3 in the same direction as pH
  PCO_2 low, HCO_3 low
C: Check compensation
Resp: acute: PCO_2 increase 10-HCO_3 increase 1-PH reduce 0.08
  Chronic: PCO_2 increase 10-HCO_3 increase 3– PH reduce 0.03
  Metab: compensate: HCO_3 increase 1-PCO_2 increase 1
D: Check anio Gap: Na-(Cl+HCO_3). Normal 12±2
  High AG: Etiology MUDPILES – Methanol, Uremia, Diabetes-
  DKA, Paraldehyde, Isopropyl alcohol, Lactate,
  Ethanol-ethylene glycerol, Salicyate.
  Normal AG: Etiology – hypoalbuminemia, renal-RTA,
  GI-fistula, ileal loop
E. Treat underlying cause, bicarb-controversial

21. Elevated Liver Enzymes, Jaundice

Case 1.

50 YOM comes to your office, mad, because his insurance turned him down for abnormal LFTs. He wants you to "sort out this mistake." Transaminase very high, ALP slightly up. Normal bilirubin, Hx, 3DDx, 2 Investigation

(Hx: heavy drinker, hetero-sexual, single partner but promiscus in youth, no contact with hepatitis, on no Meds, no street drugs, no change in stool or urine)

Key:

Possible causes include viral hepatitis, toxic/drug induced hepatitis; Alcoholic hepatitis; other tumor, trauma, etc

Hx:

- *When was the blood test done?*
- *Symptoms:*
  Do you have fever, malgia, fatigue, headache, cough, N/V, anorexia, abdominal discomfort, changes in sense of taste and smell, itching, jaundice, bruising?
  Are these symptoms getting worse/better?
- *Cause:*
  Have you had blood transfusion recently?
  Do you drink alcohol, how much?
  Are you taking any Meds such as acetaminophen, INH, methyldopa, steroids, erythromycin, etc?
  Recent travel to endemic area, contact with people with hepatitis?
  Are you living with a male/female partner? Does your partner have hepatitis or using street drugs?
  Recent serious illness/trauma?
  Have you had vaccination against Hepatitis?
  Any weight loss?
- *Previous investigation/treatment?*

PE

General:
– Malnutrition; pallor (anemia); jaundice; breath fetor
– Xanthelasmata (chronic cholestasis)
– Parotid swelling (alcohol abuse)
– Bruising, spider nevi
– Female distribution of body hair

Mental:
– Wernicke: a. ophthalmoplegia, nystagmous, ataxia, lateral rectus palsy
  b. altered mental state
– Karsakoff: a. retrograde amnesia, impaired learning
  b. confabulation

Hand:
– Flapping tremor, inability to copy a five point star
– leukonychia – hypoproteinemia
– Palmer erythema
– Mild finger clubbing, muscle atrophy

Chest:
– Gynecomastia
– Right side pleural effusion

Abdomen:
– Dilated veins, collateral
– Liver + spleen enlargement
– Ascites
– Testicular atrophy

DDx:

Viral hepatitis
Alcohol – steatohepatitis
Drugs hepatitis

Investigation

Serology: AST>ALT alcohol, ALT>AST Viral
        HbsAg, HbeAg, Anti-HbsAg, Anti-HBcAg, AntiHBeAg
        LFTs bilirubin, albumen, PTT INR
Liver biopsy, U/S, CT

Case 2.
44 YOF, presented with jaundice, take a focused history.

Hx
- *Have you travelled to areas where hepatitis A is endemic?*
- *How much alcohol do you drink per day?*
- *Have you ever used IV drugs?*
- *Ever have blood transfusion? What is your sexual orientation?*
- *Ever contacted with jaundiced patients?*
- *Have you experienced skin itching? colicky belly pain?*
- *What Meds have you taken recently?*
- *Have you have occupational contact with hepatotoxins?*
- *Do you have pain or recent weight loss?*
- *What color are your stools and urine?*
- *Is there anyone in your family with liver disease?*

22. Lower GI Bleeding

Case 1.
20 YOF maroon stools, take Hx. DDx, tests.

Case 2.
30 YOM with abdominal pain, lower GI bleeding, Bp 80/50 in distress. Give orders to the nurse in the ER.

Hx:
- *Is there a past hx of abdominal pain or other GI symptoms?*
- *Hx of chronic excessive alcohol intake?*
- *Past hx of hematemesis, melana or anemia?*
- *Are you taking any NSAIDs, steroids or other meds?*
- *Was the bleeding proceded by intense retching?*
- *Have you been taking iron pills or bismuth? R/o pseudo-bleeding*
- *Do you have liver disease?*
- *R/O severe bleeding emergency: Do you feel dizzy, SOB, light headed?*

DDx:
Local:
  Massive: diverticulosis, angiodysplasia.
  Less common: UGI, aorta-enteric fistula
  Intermittent: hemorrhoid, colitis, and anorectal lesion
  Occult: neoplasm, colon Ca
Systemic:
  Blood dyscrasia, thrombocytopenia
  Coagulation disorder (DIC)
  Vascular malformation, Vasculitis
Always ask upper GI bleed
Hematemesis:
  1). Esophageal: liver cirrhosis, alcohol, hepatitis, bruising
  2). Stomach ulcer: Aspirin, ASAID, steroids, alcohol, ulcer Hx
  3). Gastritis: trauma, burn, infection
  4). Mallory Weiss syndrome

No-Hematemesis:

1. Inflammatory bowel disease: diarrhea, urgency, Tenesmus, LQ cramping

2. Diverticulosis: brisk, frank bleeding

3. Ca: weight loss, BM habit change

Manage

- In severe case, ABCs Stablize, see upper GI bleeding
- Definitive treatment:

Sigmoidoscopy on unprepared bowel:

Diagnostic: bleeding hemorrhoids, colitis, structural lesion-treat accordingly

Non-diagnostic – Hospitalize, then

a. If bleeding stopped, clean bowel, clonoscopy

b. Bleeding <0.5 ml/min-RBC scan, Bleeding>0.5ml/min-angiogram

23. Vomiting, Constipation, Diarrhea

Case 1.
Adult patient presented with vomiting, or constipation, or chronic diarrhea, take focused history.

Case 2.
27 years old with diarrhea for 3 months, take Hx and consult.

Hx for Vomiting
- *Is the vomiting worse in the morning?*
- *Does the vomiting occur in association with meals?*
- *Is there associated abdominal pain? headache?*
- *Is the vomitus bloody or bile stained?*
- *Are there recognizable food or coffee grounds in the vomit?*
- *What drugs are being taken?*
- *Do you feel thirsty? How much do you urinate over 24 hours?*

Hx for Constipation
- *What is your normal stool frequency?*
- *Do you strain at stool?*
- *How long have you been constipated?*
- *Is there associated abdominal pain, n/v, distension?*
- *Are the stools large or small and pellet shaped?*
- *Have you noticed intercurrent diarrhea (spurious)?*
- *Are any constipating drugs, such as codeine or other opiates being used?*
- *spinal injury, surgery, tumor*

Hx for diarrhea in adult patient
Confirm Dx and assess severity
- *What is your normal stool frequency?*
- *How many stools daily? Volume?*
- *How long have you had diarrhea?*
- *Are you awakened with a bowel movement at night?*
- *What is the color and consistency of stool? Are blood, pus or mucous present?*

- *Are there associated n/v, weight loss or pain?*
- *Do you feel thirsty, dizzy? How frequent do you urinate?*

Search for etiology:
THOSE FADS WILT
Travel, Homosexual, Outbreak, Seafood, Extraintestinal
   (arthralgia, choleangitis, skin lesion, eye, thrombophlebitis)
Family history, Antibiotics, Diet, Steatorrhea
Weight loss, Immunosuppressed, Laxative use, Tumor

- *Any travel abroad? Contact with diarrhea patients? eating out?*
- *What is your sexual orientation? Unprotected anal sex?*
- *Any purgative/laxative abuse?*
- *Any antibiotics or other meds?*
- *Are you under stress or anxious for something?*
- *Is the diarrhea related with eating in a timely fashion (irritable bowel Syndrome)?*
- *Associate symptoms:*
  Periumbilical/RLQ pain/copious watery stool – small bowel
  LLQ pain/tenesmus/frequent small volume – large bowel
  Macular rose spot, rash on trunk – typhoid
  Fever, blood, pus – invasive, tumor, infection by invasive bacteria like shigella
  Joint, eye symptoms – inflammatory bowel disease
  Mucus free of leukocyte, alter solid/soft-irritable bowel syndrome
  Diarrhea follows meals-malabsorption, dumping syndrome, fistula
  Foul bulky greasy – fat malabsorption
  Frothy stool, excessive flatus – fermentation of unabsorbed carbohydrate
  Previous gastrectomy – dumping syndrome

Patient education for diarrhea:
Encourage take fluids, won't make diarrhea worse
Sugar and juice will make it worse
Kaolin-pectin, no effect, no harm
Antibiotics-resistant strains/complications/side effects
Bismuth (Pepto-Bismol) for emergency use, effective
Advise bottled water

Undiagnosed, chronic-need extensive evaluation

Personal hygiene: sitz bath absorbed cotton, barrier cream

Recovery phase; avoid milk/dairy products for 7 days because mild lactase intolerance, use easy digested food banana, rice, bake potato

Chapter 3. Obstetrics and Gynecology

Menstrual History

- *Age of menarche, telarche?*
- *Use of BCP or HRT?*
- *Length of cycle? Days of blood loss? Number of tampons or pads used per day?*
- *Are there clots?*
- *Has there been a change in the periodicity of your cycle?*

Obstetric History

- *Have you ever been pregnant? If so, how often?*
- *Did you have any problems getting pregnant?*
- *How many children do you have?*
- *Have you miscarried, and if so, at what stage of pregnancy?*
- *Were there any complications in pregnancy? Like HTN, DM*
- *Was the labor normal or did you require forceps or C-section?*

1. Amenorrhea

Case 1.

30 YOF presents with ammenorrhea. Dehydroepiandrosterone
sulfate (DHEAS) elevated, LH normal and prolactin normal. Obtain a
focused history and manage.
Diagnosis: Ovarian failure
Q: She wants to get pregnant, what can you do?

Keys:

Primary ammenorrhea: if pubic and axillary hair growth, breast
development, and female voice have commenced. Investigate
only after age 16.

Secondary Amenorrhea: Cessation of menses for 3 or more
months in a patient with previous normal cycles.

History:

- *How many periods have you actually missed?*
- *Were your periods regular before? How irregular?*
- *Is this the first time you period stopped? Did it suddenly stop?*
- *When do you start not having a period? LMP*
- *Any stress, depression, bereavement? Any changes of living environment?*
- *Are you afraid of getting pregnant?*
- *Do you think you might be pregnant?*
  Any milk comes out of the breast? – do you have n/v in the morning
  – urine frequency – tender enlarged breast?
- *How much exercise do you do? Have you lost any weight? -Anorexia*
  nervosa
- *Notice any change in your body? Voice, hair?*
- *Are you taking any Meds-BCP?*
- *How old are you? Do you have hot flashes, dryness of introitus and*
  vagina?
- *Do you have smell/vision changes? breast discharge? headache? libido?*
  – pituitary, hypothalmus
- *How do you like the cold weather? – hypothroidism*
- *PMHx: obstetric/gyne/menstrual/sex, AMPLE*

- *FHx: Are your mother/sister's period normal at this age?*

Management.
In sequence:
1. Focused physical exam: appearance: cachexia/obesity, cushings, hirsutism, vision, breast, vagina, (ovarian, adenexual), adrenal
2. Pregnancy test
3. TSH and prolactin
4. Progesterone challenge: withdrawl bleed (+)anovulation, (-)end organ failure
5. LH, FSH
- In + withdrawl bleeding, LH high – polycystic ovary, LH low – hypothalamic
- In - withdrawl bleeding, FSH high-ovary failure
  FSH low, hypothalmic or pituitary
6. DHEA, testosterone high: polycystic ovary, ovary androgen secreting tumor, adrenal tumor, late onset 21-hydroxylase deficiency

Patient education:
1. Cope with stress
2. BCP, not been rendered infertile. Normal period will resume in 6 months time,
3. If don't want to be pregnant, use barrier method, because spontaneous ovulation
4. If patient wants to get pregnant:
   Clomephene
   Human menopausal gonadotropin (HMG)
   Traditional bilateral ovary wedge resection
5. Need to work out the cause, not wait and see. Don't want to miss a serious illness.

2. Menorrhagia

Case 1.
42 YOF heavy vaginal bleeding for the last 3 periods. Hx. Dx. Manage

Keys:
1. Diagnostic criteria: Menstrual period >80 ml or> 7 days
2. Anovulatory bleeding occurs at two age extremes: either very young (menarche) or old (starting menopause)

History:
- *How old are you?*
- *What is your current and previous pattern of menstrual bleeding, length, duration, volume?*
- *When did it start to change? gradual or suddenly, any suspected cause?*
- *Timing: when exactly the bleeding occurs, intermenstrual/postcoital?*
- *Any change in the pattern or volume? Getting worse/better?*
- *Associated symptoms:*

Sx of anemia: dizzy, black out, palpation, BP dropping
Sx of infection: fever, discharge, dysuria, dysparunia, abdomial pain
Sx of malignancy: weight loss
Sx of endocrine abnormality
   Hirsutism – voice change, hair pattern change, fat distribution
   Galactorrhea – any dischage from breast?
   Hypothyroidism: slow movements, heat/cold intolerance, constipation
Sx of pregnancy, pregnancy complications.
Pelvic pain-infection, adenomyosis, degenerated fibroid
- *Sexual/OB-Gy STD BCP history*
- *Premenstrual molimina (ovulation), any mood changes?*
- *Bruising, excessive bleeding at other sites.*
- *Any previous investigations?*

PMHx: *kidney, liver, coagulation disorder, diabetes, obesity, hypothyroidism, pelvic pathology*
Meds: *contraceptive, steroids, phenothiazines*

DDx:

Polyps, leomyoma

Endometrial hyperplasia/Ca

Endometriosis/adenomyosis

Infection/STD

Chronic anovulation, estrogen withdrawl

Menopausal

Non-Gyne: coagulopathy, liver disease, SLE, hypothyroidism

Manage:

- Investigations: CBC PTT INR, LH, FSH, PRH, TSH, pregnancy test, hysteroscopy, D+C, U/S endometrial biopsy, PV, pap smear
- Anemia: Iron, foliac acid supplement, transfusion
- Oral contraception pill, progesterone support
- D+C
- Treat etiology

3. Vaginal Bleeding, General, First and Second Trimester

Case 1.

42 YOF female presents with per vaginal (PV) bleeding. Obtain a history. What is your differential diagnosis and investigation plan?

Key:

Rule out etiologies other than dysfunctional uterine bleeding.

History:

- *Onset: How much blood? (Pads/tampons use). Tissue/clots noticed? Smell?*
- *Abdominal cramps/pain? Fever?*
- *Severity? Changes over time? Aggravation/relieve factors?*
- *How is you normal menstrual period? Regularity, amounts? Intermenstrual period?*
- *How does this compare to your normal period?*
- *LMP? Obstetric, pregnancy, delivery, abortion/Gyne, STD, BCP*
- *Possibility of pregnancy: Unprotected sex, breast engorgement, fatigue, urine frequency, N/V*
- *Sx of malignancy: Postcoital bleeding, fever, weight loss*
- *Sx of anemia: dizziness, SOB, black out?*
- *Sx of STD: belly pain, fever, vaginal discharge, urine frequency, and dyspareunia*
- *PMHx: AMPLE, drink smoke, STD, Pap smear*
- *Bleeding diathesis, meds inhibit normal clotting*
- *Other: stress, exercise, chronic illness, diet, hirsutism, infertility, obesity*

Differential Diagnosis:

Ovulatory: Normal variant, anatomic lesion, fibroid, tumor, bleeding diathesis, IUD

Anovulatory: BCP, breakthrough, hypothalamic stress, and polycystic ovary

Postmenopausal: Tumor, fibroid, polyp, inflammation, pills

Pregnancy: Abortion, ectopic pregnancy, molar pregnancy

Management of Dysfuctional Uterine Bleeding (DUB):

- ABC, vitals
- CBC, type and cross, blood gas, pregnancy test, PTT, INR, LFTs
- Vit K, transfusion
- Estrogen
- By cyclic progestin therapy from day 14 to 25 of each cycle or
- By daily combination oral contraceptive pill (OCP)
- Angiography, embolization
- Surgery

Case 2.

7 weeks into her pregnancy, a lady presents with vaginal bleeding and lower abdominal pain. She has had a previous abortion at 6 wks. Obtain a focused history in 5 minutes. What is your diagnosis, differential diagnosis, management plan and investigation?

Key:

Try to identify the cause of a repeated abortion.

History:

- *Cramping pains, fever?*
- *Purulent discharge?*
- *Do you still feel the baby is alive?*
- *Have you had previous first trimester bleeding?*
- *Have you had tissue pass through the birth canal?*
- *Have you had an U/S to locate the position of the placenta?*
- *Any previous uterine surgery?*
- *Any coagulation abnormalities in the past?*
- *Any use of tobacco or illicit drugs?*

Differential Diagnosis and Management:

1. Abortion:
   a. Threatened: U/S viability of fetus
   b. Incomplete or inevitable: D&C +/- Oxytocin
   c. Complete: No Tx

     d. Septic: D/C+ antibiotic+ oxygen
2. Ectopic pregnancy – surgery
3. Molar pregnancy – surgery, chemo
4. Cervical polyp, genital Ca – surgery
5. Physiological bleeding (placental development) – supportive, observation

Investigations:

1. Speculum examination is essential to rule out vaginal or cervical lesions that are causing bleeding
2. Molar and ectopic pregnancy should be ruled out in all patients with early pregnancy bleeding (so:U/S, BhCG testing)
3. Cytogenetic (Turner Syndrome), Mendelian etiology (autosomal or X-linked dominant or recessive diseases)
4. Anticardiolipin antibody test

4. Vaginal Discharge

Case 1.
60 YOF with bloody vaginal discharge. Obtain a history.

Case 2.
19 YOF with 5-day vaginal discharge. Obtain a history and provide 3 differential diagnoses, 2 simple investigations and 3 lines of advice.

Key:
Smell, color and timing are important.

History:
- *How long has the discharge been present? Acute / chronic, new/ old?*
- *Is the discharge scanty or profuse?*
- *Is extra protection necessary or does the discharge simply spot or stain?*
- *What is the color and consistency? Is it sticky or cheesy?*
- *Is there an odor?*
- *Is the discharge blood-stained?*
- *Any change in characteristics recently?*
- *Timing? When does the discharge usually happen? Post-coital, mid-cycle*
- *Is there associated abdominal pain or a fever?*
- *Is there itching or burning of the vulvar area?*
- *Do you experience pain or a burning sensation when you urinate? How many times do you have to get up to urinate at night?*
- *Do you have pain or discomfort when you have sexual intercourse?*
- *Have you noticed any skin rashes?*
- *Have you had unprotected sexual intercourse? Discharge in partner?*
- *Hygiene: bubble bath, genital deodorants, soaps, use of wipers, douching habits, clothing habits (underwear),*
- *Weight loss, cough, bone pain (low back)*
- *Sex/ menstrual / OB-GYN, BCP, use of pad, tampon, IUD, drugs, alcohol,*
- *AMPLE: previous vaginal infection, diabetes, and use of antibiotics/ steroids*

2 investigations:
- Vaginal secretions for culture and sensitivity, saline wet mount, KOH wet mount, pH.
- Smear microscopy, Gram stains

Differential Diagnosis:
1. **Infectious:**
   STD: gonorrhea, herpes, chlamydia, trichomonas, PID
   Non-STD: Candida, bacteria (gardnerella)
2. **Physiologic hormonal change:** Leukorrhea, atrophic vaginitis
3. Other: chemical, allergic, foreign body, IUD, Ca, polyp, cervicitis

Advice and Treatment:
- *Hygiene: avoid nylon underwear, panty hose, wet-bathing suits, tight jeans, allergens*
- *Safer sex*
- *Complete treatment and treat partner, avoid sex during treatment.*
- *Gardnerella vaginalis ⇒ Ampicillin. If pregnant ⇒ Flagyl 500 mg Bid*
- *Trichomonas vaginalis ⇒ Flagyl*
- *Chlamydia trachomatis ⇒ Doxycycline 100 mg Bid*
- *Candida' ⇒ Fluconazol cream or oral anti-fungal medications*

5. Pregnancy at Old Age, Counselling

Case 1.
37 YOF, G1 P0, 9 weeks pregnant. Manage.

Key:
- Risks of complications, esp. Down's syndrome
- Explain prenatial screening program: when to start, what can be done

History:
- *How old are you? Is this your first pregnancy?*
- *Is this a planed pregnancy? Is this your first visit?*
- *When was your LMP? Do you have any symptoms like fatigue, N/V, backache, groin pain, constipation?* Confirm pregnancy, determine gestational age, expected delivery date (EDD) = LMP+7day-3month
- * *Medical history: Are you healthy? Do you have any serious illness like diabetes, heart, liver, kidney, HTN?*
- *Obstetrical history of all previous pregnancies: GTPA L/year sex/weight/gestational age/mode of delivery/length of labor/ complications/uterine surgery (myomectomy. D+C, cone biopsies).*
- *Family history of genetic disease? AMPLE*
- *Is there any thing you are especially worrying about at this point? Family support? Body image, libido, need for security, illness?*
- *Is there a history of contact with infectious disease during pregnancy?*
- *How do you feel about becoming a mother? How does your husband feel?*

Consult:
- There is an increased risk of Down's syndrome and other abnormalities because of the mother's age at pregnancy (age 20 1:2000, age 30 1:900, age 35 1:365, age 40 1:110, age 45 1:30, age 47 1:20).
  Screening tests available:
  10-12 wk chroionic villi sampling (CVS)
  12-16 wk amniocentesis

16wk MSS (MSAFP, hcG, uE3) Trisomy 18 all low, Downs hcG high, other two low

16-18wk U/S,

26-28 wk 50g OGCT,

28wk repeat CBC, Rhogam to Rh(-) mother,

36 RhAb screen, GBS screen

Risks of CVS or amniocentesis are 1% abortion, infection, bleeding, etc. What should she do? Go home and discuss with husband. Perform procedures only if the information will alter her approach to the pregnancy based on the results.

- Several things should be avoided: irradiation, X-ray, smoking, alcohol, cat litter, drugs, hot tub/sauna, infection like rubella (fever), HIV, varicellat

- Several things you can have: sex, regular exercise

- Several things you need to have: Nutrition with added Ca^{2+}, iron, folic acid, Vitamin B12, appropriate weight gain. (expect to gain 1 lb per month in the first half of pregnancy, 1 lb per week in the 2nd half. Average 25-35 lbs with only 40% from conception)

- For women who do not consume an adequate diet, a daily multivitamin should be continued in the second trimester

- Danger signs: Bleeding, cramping (contraction), dysuria, vaginitis, weight loss

  Mention: other risks of high maternal age: pre-eclampsia/eclampsia, chronic HTN, obesity, DM, fibroids

Documentation:
- Weight, baseline BP
- ABO Rh, Hb
- Rubella Ab
- VDRL, HIV, HbsAg
- MSU
- Electrophoresis for abnormal Hb in women of Africa, Indian, Mediterranean
- Pelvic Exam: Pap smear, culture for GC/chlamydia
- Are you planning to give birth here? Is everything arranged at home? work?

- Schedule visit every 4 wk until 28 wk, then
  every 2 wk until 36 wk, then
  every 1 wk until delivery

Unwanted Pregnancy, Counselling

Case 1.

24 YOF, pregnant, she doesn't want to give birth to a child at this time in her life. Provide consult.

Keys:

1. Confirm diagnosis,
2. Inform the patient about community service available for prenatal care: abortion, adoption, motherhood

How does she feel about the pregnancy? Does she want to carry to term? If so, will she keep the baby? If she wants an abortion, then go through the following. If she wants to keep the baby, manage and counsel as for an expectant mother.

Confirm Diagnosis:

You are pregnant, is that right?
How do you know that?
What symptoms you have? Any pregnancy test? Ultrasound?
How far along is the pregnancy?
This is an unplanned pregnancy, is that right?

Counsel

Are there any special reasons you don't want to keep this child?
Do you have financial difficulty?
Do you think that having a baby might affect you opportunity of education/ career advancement?
Do you have chronic or serious illness? Diabetes, cancer, HIV?
Are you using drugs, alcohol, or smoking?
Are you a high school student? Teenager?
Are you worried about the possible genetic abnormalities?
Did this pregnancy happen as a result of rape or sexual abuse?
How do you feel about becoming a mother?
What is your initial thought when you started to know that your are pregnant?

What is your opinion about abortion? Before? Now?

How does your partner feel about this? How does your family feel about this?

What do you want to do with this pregnancy?

Are you aware of the **options** *we have?*

The options are:

A. Therapeutic abortion:

   Medical: <9w methotrexate+misprotol (EXP.)

   >12w prostaglandin intra/extra amniotically, or IM

   Surgical: 12-16W D+C >16w D+evacuation

   Complication (0.1%) include: perforation, infection, sterility, cervix laceration, asherman's Sx

B. Adoption

C. Keep the child

How much do you know about abortion?

Procedure and risks?

- Procedure: Lie on a table, general anesthesia, suction through cervix.
- Risks: uterus perforation 0.1%, major hemorrhage 0.06% unless you have coagulation disorder, cervical laceration 0.1-1%, delayed bleeding or retained placenta, infection.
- No obvious effect on subsequent pregnancies except after a late abortion where forceful cervical dilation occurs

When do you want it to be done?

What contraceptive method have you been using?

What method are you planning to use in the future?

I would like to see you after the procedure to discuss your feelings and concerns afterwards.

7. Pre-eclampsia, Eclampsia, Manage

Case 1.
36 wks gestation, proteinuria + BP 130/85 (from 110/65), Manage.

Case 2.
36 wks pregnancy with increasing swelling of feet and hands. BP 140/80 at 16 wks pregnancy. Counsel and manage.

Diagnostic criteria:
Pre-eclampsia:
Hypertension+ proteinuria and/or non-dependent edema at >20 wks pregnancy.

Systolic blood pressure increased 30 or diastolic blood pressure increased 15 or >140/90
- mild: no neurological Sx or the following criteria
- severe: BP>160/100 with CVS-heart failure; Renal–elevated serum CT, oligouria, proteinuria >2+ or > 5g/24hr; Liver-ascites, elevated liver enzyme and bilirubin; Nervous system – headache, visual disturbances, clonus.

Eclampsia: Pre-eclampsia+seizure

Manage:
- Mild Pre- eclampsia
- Maternal evaluation: Hx, PE, CBC lytes, urine analysis, PTT INR, FDP, LFTs, 24 hr urine, Cr-clearance, protein
- Fetal evaluation: FHR, NST, BPP
- Rest, left decubitus position.
- Normal diet, no Meds

- Severe pre-eclampsia
Stabilize and deliver
- Admit, IV, cross match blood, urine catheter, NPO
- Evaluation and Monitor
Mother: vitals, input/output, DTR, urine protein
Fetus: NST electronic

- Anticonvulsant. Mg Sulfate 4g IV push – 2-4g/hr
- Anti-hypertensive: Hydrolazine 5-10mg IV push over 5 min, q30min.
- Continue post-partum management for at least 24 hr until stablized.

- Eclampsia
- ABCs
- Control seizure
- Complication: lung aspiration, acidosis, fracture.

Do not try to shorten or abolish initial convulsion, prevent injury to mother and maintain adequate oxygenation

8. Pregnancy, Abdominal Pain

Case 1.
25 YOF, pregnant, LLQ pain. a). Perform physical exam, b). Important history points, c). Investigations, d). 3DDx

a. Physical exam:
- Vitals, BP sitting and supine, look for signs of bleeding (pale, shock).
- Abdomen:
   Inspection-surgical scar, shape
   Palpation-pain, mass, rebound tenderness
   Percussion-fluid (blood), uterus span
   Auscultation-bowel sound, fetus heart beat, etc
- Gynecological exam

b. Important history points: Any bleeding? How many wks gestation? Feel baby moving anymore? Risk factors for abruption-vascular disease, HTN, pre-eclampsia, cocaine, previous abruptio, trauma

c. Investigation: Mother– U/S, CBC, PTT, INR
   Fetus-non-stress test, heart rate, biophysical profile (BPP) by U/S.

d. DDx: Ectopic preg. Placenta abruptio, placenta previa, abortion, ovarian cyst (hyperreactio luteinalis)

9. Breast Feeding, Counselling

Case 1.
29 YOF, pregnant, has concerns about breast feeding, provide consult.

Key:
nutrition, absorption, immune (IgG, IgA), bond.

- Breast milk suits infant's immature GI tract, kidney, immune system and metabolic demands.
- Nutrition: 50% energy from Fat, contains essential FFA, 90% absorption; Low protein than Cow's milk, low renal load but more essential AAs; higher whey content (easy digested protein) less casein; 50% Fe absorption vs 10% absorption of Cow's milk.
- Breast milk contains IgA, macrophages, active lymphocytes, lysozyme; promote growth of lactobacillus in GI
- Breast milk is less allergen
- Psychosocial bonding, economic
- Contraindications for breast feeding: HIV/AIDS; active untreated TB; regional herpes; using alcohol/drug; chemo/radioactive therapy

10. C- section, Counselling

Case 1.

20 YOF, pregnant, has had a C-section with 1st baby due to fetal distress. Counsel fears of 2nd C-section.

Key:

Address patient's concerns directly, pain, future delivery, and cosmetic.

History:

Hx and general consult same as counseling an unwanted pregnancy.

- *Tell me more about last pregnancy?*
- *Why the decision of C-section?*
- *Why are you worried about 2nd C-section?*
- *Any complications/discomfort last time?*
- *Any problems with social support?*
- *Do you have the same risk factors as last time?*

Consult:

- Most people can a have successful vaginal delivery after a C-section, even after 2 C-sections.
- Particularly in low-transverse incision.
- In classical vertical incision, vaginal delivery is not encouraged because of risks of uterine rupture.
- We'll arrange to admit you as soon as you are in labor, closely monitor both you and the child, and we will attempt vaginal delivery first.
- If a 2nd C-section is needed, the operation is still very safe. If you wish to have a C-section anyway, we can schedule you, too.

11. Birth Control Counselling

Case 1.
21 YOF is requesting birth control pills (BCP). Counsel.

Key:
Explain the risks and benefits of available methods and answer
the patient's questions. You need to ask about the patient's
obs/gyn/sex history before addressing the BCP subject.

History:
Imagine this scenario:
- *Hi, I am Dr. X. I am here to provide you with some information about
  BCP. Is this the first time you are using them? Yes*
- *Well, they are safe pills IF you:*
  Are not older than 35
  Do not smoke
  Are not pregnant
  Do not have: (contraindications)
      1. Vaginal bleeding
      *2. Coronary/cerebral vascular disease; HTN, thromboembolic
         events*
      3. Estrogen-dependent tumor in breast, liver or uterus
      4. Impaired liver function
      5. Congenital hyperlipidemia
- *Do you have any of these conditions?*

Consult:
- BCP are very effective with a failure rate of 1%
- However, it cannot protect you from STD's.
- I must warn you that these pills are hormones and can:
      Have estrogenic effects:
      Worsen migraines
      Worsen seizures
      Increase body weight
      Elevate blood pressure
      Aggravate uterine fibroma

Cause gestational DM

Have progesterone effects:

Cause depression

Cause acne

Cause hirsutism

How do I use them?

- Start the 1st pill on Day 1 of your cycle. It takes time for the meds to work. You will need to use barrier methods during the first month.

What happens if I miss a pill?

- Take 2 pills if you remember the 2nd day
- Use Condoms at the same time
- Another thing I want to mention is if you ...
o   Have vomiting
o   Have diarrhea
o   Are taking certain antibiotics like rifampin or phenobarb
BCP may not work well.
- On the other hand, BCP can also alter the effects of other meds. Check with you doctor each time you are put on new meds.

Explain the anatomy and the reproductive cycle
Take a brief Hx of sexual/menstrual/OB-Gyn

- *I will keep the information you give me confidential. Are you aware of other methods?*

BCP:

- Mechanism:
  Estrogen: inhibits ovulation, speeds egg movement
  Progestin: makes cervical mucous thicker, vicious, inhibits endometrium proliferation
- Risks, benefits and contraindications: See above.

Other methods:

Physiologic method:

- Rhythm, coitus interruptus
- Require significant motivation by couples, regular menses
- Still need back-up method such as condom
- Failure rate 4-5%, no side effect

Surgical Methods:
Tube sterilization
        Vasectomy, failure 0.1-0.2%
Barrier Methods:
Condom:
  Benefits: effective, 3% failure, protects against STD, handy
  Risks: interrupts love making, breaks, care during withdrawal
Diaphragm:
  Benefits: Easy, may protect against STD
  Risks: 6% failure, possible UTI, must fit, use jelly/cream, remain
  6-8 hrs after intercourse
Vaginal sponge:
  Benefits: Easy, may protect against STD
  Risks: 6-9% failure, TSS, remove intact
Vaginal chemicals, foams, cream, jelly, suppository:
  Benefits: easy, may protect against STD
  Risks: 3% failure, allergies, messy, inconvenient

Intra-Uterine Device (IUD):
  IUD are made of flexible plastic, some wrapped with copper or
  progesterone. Those with copper need to be replaced every 5
  years to prevent infection with actinomycosis.
Mechanism: stimulate inflammatory response to lyse blast,
  interfere with endometrial proliferation
Benefits: effective, 1% failure, convenient
Risks: cramping, mid-cycle bleeding, heavy periods, ectopic
  pregnancy, PID, infertility, perforation, expulsion
Progesterone implant/injection:
- Benefits: effective, 0.01% failure, convenient
- Risks: spotting, irregular/absent menses, weight gain

12. Infertility

Case 1.

32 YOF, married for 5 years, infertility. Obtain a focused history in 5 minutes.

- *How long have you been married or living with your current partner? How long have you been trying to have a child?*
- *Have you ever been pregnant? – details*
- *What birth control methods have you ever used?*
- *How often do you have sexual intercourse? Do you use creams or lubricants with intercourse?*
- *Have you had any investigation procedure for fertility?*
- *Do you have kidney, bladder, vaginal infection? STD?*
- *Do you drink, smoke, use street drugs or on any meds?*
- *Do you have DM, thyroid disease, heart disease, RA or any other medical condition?*
- *Do you notice any discharge from your breast?*
- *How about your period? menarche, menopause, regular or not?*
- *Have your weight been stable over the last 2 years?*
- *When was your last pap smear? how was it?*
- *Anybody in your family had difficulty getting pregnant?*

Chapter 4. Pediatrics

Approach to Infants

History:
- *Feeding hx, birth weight*
- *Maternal health, pregnancy and delivery*
- *Vitamin K administration, iron supplement*
- *Jaundice, stools, wet diapers*
- *How does he/she respond to handling?*
- *Immunization updated?*

Assess Development:
Gross motor, fine motor
Vision, hearing
Expressive language, comprehension
Social skills, behavior

1. Hematolytic-uremic Sydrome

Case 1.
Child with HUS, bloody stool. Obtain a history

Key:
HUS triad – Nephropathy, microangiopathic thrombocytopenia, and hemolytic anemia

History:
- *Did he have any contact with animals, especially cattle or young calves (e.g., by a major reservoir)?*
- *Any contact with animal manure used as fertilizer? They can contaminate produce (potatoes, lettuce, fallen apples).*
- *When did this start? Suddenly/gradually?*
- *Did he catch a cold? Cough, fever?*
- *Travel recently? Anybody close (e.g., in daycare) having the same problem?*
- *What did you eat before that?*
- *Eaten hamburger in the last week (5-7 days E.coli toxin H157)?*
- *How much blood in the stool? Do you feel lightheaded?*
- *What does the stool look like? Bright red, dark?*
- *Do you have fever, belly pain? Tenesmus?*
- *Any change in urine? Oligouria, Hematuria*
- *Any skin rashes? Where? Is it very itchy?*
- *Do you have weight loss?*
- *Do you have bleeding somewhere else? Epistaxis, bruise, Hematuria?*
- *How has your blood pressure been?*
- *Any mood change? (Irritable)*
- *AMPLE*

2. Febrile Seizure
Case 1.
Lady whose 18 month old had seizure. Obtain a history and describe the character of febrile seizures as well as the risk of recurrence.

Case 2.
8 month old with febrile seizures. What do you do and what do you tell the parents?

Key:
Determine whether the event was truly a seizure.

History:
- *Hi, I am Dr. X. What is wrong with Aaron?*
  He was shaking, I was very worried, So I brought him over.
- *Is this the first time? Yes*
- *When does the shaking started? How long does it last? 2 minutes*
- *What did you do? I took him to the washroom into a cool water tub, since sponging was not good.*
- *Did he have a fever? How high was the temperature? Yes, See he had a fever for 2 days.*
- *Any relatives having similar Sx? Yes, His dad had these when he was young.*
- *What Sx does he have during the seizure? (type of seizure, local/general?)*
- *Are there any epileptogenic factors such as prior head trauma, stroke, etc.?*
- *Is there any underlying CNS disease?* A careful assessment of developmental milestones may provide evidence for underlying CNS disease.
- *Are there are any precipitating factors such as sleep deprivation, systemic disease, electrolyte or metabolic derangements, acute infection, drugs that lower the seizure threshold etc.?*
- *Does it cause any body damage? Tongue biting, fractures, urine incontinence?*
- *What happened after the seizure? Is there any neurological defect after seizure?*
- *Prenatal, delivery, Apgar at delivery, development, head trauma, meningitis*

- *Is he otherwise well? Any developmental/neurological problems?*

Typical febrile seizure:
- Occurs between age 6 months and 6 years of age. Temperature >39°C, or rapid rise
- Last <15min, 95%< 5min, generalized, symmetric, tonic-clonic, normal EEG
- Doesn't recur in 24 hours. No neurological defect.

Recurrence:
- General chance of recurrence is 33%.
  onset <1 yr old, 50% chance.
  onset >1yr old, 28% chance.
- If complex seizure of previous abnormal neurology exam, risk of recurrence is higher
- Risk of epilepsy is 5%

Suggest: Tylenol, tepid sponging, cold bath, prevent accidents, mark intervals

Q: Will this Sx recur? Yes, 33% of the time.

Q: Will he grow out of it? Yes, by the age 6-8.

Q: What are 3 clues in hx indicate febrile seizure?

- *Age, duration and fever-related*

Q: What directions would you give Mom about what to do?

  Tepid bath, tylenol, put on soft bed, avoid damage

3. Physical Abuse

Case 1.
Obtain a history and provide a consult regarding physical abuse.

Case 2.
Father abuses child, -consult mom.

Key:
Interview child and parents separately.
Assess whether injury on PE correlates with history provided.

History:
- *What, when, how, why happened to this child? Are there any other children at home?*
- *Is there any clinical/unexplained injury? For example 2 month old baby rolled over from the sofa and fell.*
- *To mother:*
  What do you do when he/she cries?
  Who lives with you at home? What does your husband do when the child cries?
  Any job, financial problems? Under any stress? Was this pregnancy planned?
  Do you or your husband use drugs, alcohol?
  Were you or your husband abused as a child?
  Are you or your husband suffering from any illness or psychiatric problem?
- *About the child:*
  Was he premature at birth?
  Separated from parents soon after birth?
  Handicapped or mentally retarded
  Hyperactive or difficult to discipline?
  What does he eat?
  What immunizations has he had?
  Is he in daycare or in school? How is he doing there?

Physical Exam:
- lash marks, loop marks
- bite >3 cm – adult
- Retinal hemorrhage – shaken baby
- old healing fractures, bruises
- venereal disease in prepubertal child
- Signs of neglect: dirty, FTT, malnutrition, and chronic infection
- Social isolation: apathetic
- Unexplained injury: repeated, symmetrical, instrument shape, multiple fracture, bruising above waist

Management:
- Document, REPORT
- Admit to hospital
- Report to child aid agency

4. Neonatal Jaundice

Case 1.
Female infant at 48 hours of age presented with jaundice. Obtain a history. What is your differential diagnosis, management plan and how would you advise?

Case 2.
A baby has a bilirubin of 220, normal 200, on day 2. You are asked to take a history from Mom.

Keys:
1. Rh hemolysis rarely occur in 1st baby but ABO hemolysis does
2. ABO hemolysis is mostly seen in a baby with A/B and the Mom with an O.

History:
For Mother:
* *Any disease during pregnancy? Early rupture of membrane? Maternal illness – intrauterine infection-neonatal sepsis?*
* *Do you have any thyroid problems? Did you take any pills to treat a thyroid problem during pregnancy?*
* *Do you smoke, drink, taking any Meds?*
* *Any difficulty with this delivery? Was it a vaginal delivery or a C-section?*
* *Any (scalp hematoma) or bruising?*
* *Any genetic disease runs in the family?*

For Child:
* *Is this your 1st baby?*
* *Is this child term, pre-term or post-term?*
* *How old is the baby today? What was the exact time the baby was born?*
* *How much did the baby weigh when he was born? (IUGR)*
* *Do you have any idea what his Apgar score was?*
* *How long did you and your baby stay in the hospital?*
* *When did the jaundice start? Notice any changes?*
* *Was the jaundice noticed within the first 24 hrs?*

- *Was he still jaundiced at the 3rd week of life?*
- *Does the color become more and more yellow or does it stay the same?*
- *Is the baby well otherwise? Is he breast fed? Is the baby feeding or sleeping well?*
- *Has he passed meconium? What are the color of stools and the urine?*
- *Did the baby have any bruises on the arms or a bump on the head?*
- *Do you know what the baby's blood type is? What about your own and your husband's?*
- *Do you know whether you are Rh + or -? Did you get shots during pregnancy for negative Rh?*
- *Is there anybody in your family who has a history of yellow skin?*
- *What about your other kids? Did they have yellow skin after birth?*
- *Did the baby had any blood tests done for the yellow skin?*
- *Do you know his bilirubin level?*
- *Ethnic background*

Differential Diagnosis:

1. Physiologic
- Appears >24 hours of age
- peaks at <12.9 by 3 days
- resolves by 1 week

2. Pathologic
- Appears <24 hrs of age
- Peak level >13
- Lasts > 1 wk
- If < 24hr, always pathologic: hemolysis, hemorrhage, sepsis, drugs, dehydration
- If > 3wk R/o:
  Breast milk
  Hypothyroidism
  Hepatitis
  Conjugate dysfunction, metabolism
  Impaired excretion
- In neonates, unconjugated indirect hyperbilirubinemia is predominant. Conjugated direct hyperbilirubinemia due to intra- or extra- hepatic biliary obstruction is very rare.

Bilirubin overproduction:

Hemolysis-ABO/Rh incompatibility, G-6-PD deficiency, spherocytosis

Hemorrhage-bruising, scalp hematoma

Polycythemia-IUGR

Decreased hepatic process:

Sepsis: inhibit liver enzyme

Prematurity: insufficient liver enzyme

Crigler-Najar syndrome: congenital absence of liver enzyme

Breast feeding: inhibit liver enzyme, prolonged jaundice

Hypothyroidism, Down's syndrome: low or absent liver enzyme

Increased entero-hepatic circulation:

Delayed passage of meconium (simple delay/cystic fibrosis)

Case 3.

O positive, 3rd baby. 2nd baby was jaundiced, born at term, normal delivery with no difficulty, membrane ruptured 36 hrs before delivery, breast feeding, baby well except lethargic.

Q: 1) 3 possible Dx, 2). What do you want to know about the bilirubin? 3) Investigations? 4) Immediate treatment plan?

3 Possible Diagnoses: Physiologic, sepsis, and hemolysis

About the bilirubin: direct vs. indirect, level of elevation during what time period, changes over time.

5 Lab Tests:

• LFTs, Bil-direct, indirect, HbsAg
• CBC, HB, Type, Rh antibody, coombs test
• C+S, blood, urine
• Blood smear, marrow
• U/S liver, CBD
• T4, TSH if hypothyroidism is suspected

Management:

• Observation for physiologic jaundice and breast milk induced-jaundice, breast feeding is usually not stopped

- Phototherapy + bilirubin follow-ups q6h
  a. Initiate phototherapy when:Bilirubin >300 mmol/L for a baby >2500 gm
  or Bilirubin>250 mmol/L for a baby at 2000-2500 gm
  b. Contraindicated if conjugated hyperbilirubinemia (bronzed baby)
- Hospitalization – prematurity, sepsis or severe hemolysis
- Hydration, Acid-base balance
- Exchange transfusion
- Treat underlying cause

5. Sexual Abuse

Case 1.
6 YOF, pain on micturition, suspect sexual abuse. Obtain a history from the mother.

Case 2.
Grandmother called to say the child's father is sexually abusing. Take a history; Would you tell the mother? What would you do if you suspect abuse?

Keys:
1. Child victims of sexual abuse may present with physical findings including anogenital problems, enuresis or encopresis. Behavioral changes may involve sexual acting out, aggression, depression, eating disturbances and regression.
2. Because the examination findings of most child victims of sexual abuse are within normal limits or are nonspecific, the child's statements are extremely important.
3. Get a clear picture of child and parent's behavior before, during and after an episode of abuse.

History:
- *Is this the first time she has had a UTI?*
- *When did she start having this problem?*
- *Is she sick otherwise? Fever, belly pain?*
- *What is the family situation? Has this child been left with her father, brother, uncle?*
- *How is she getting along during her day?*

- *How about her father (uncle, brother)? Does he use drugs, drink alcohol?*
- *Do you notice anything abnormal between him and this child?*
- *Has he ever abused you or the child?*

- *How is the child doing?*
- *Any sign of enuresis or encopresis?*

- *Do you notice anything abnormal regarding her:*
    Sexual knowledge
    Mood-depression
    Self-esteem
    Substance abuse
    Eating disorder
    Relationship with others

- To parent:
How is your sexual life? (Good, why? Have you heard anything?)
I received a phone call which made me suspicious? (Who was the caller?)
I'll keep it confidential for the time being, but I need to see the baby. Can you bring her over?

- *Any sibling abuse as well, how frequent UTI's?*

After Physical Exam:
- *This situation is unusual. I suspect sexual abuse.*
- *I am required by law to report this situation to the Child support agency (CSA).*
- *Do you think you and the child will be safe when you get home?*
- *Any questions?*

- If you suspect abuse:
    Examine child, document findings
    Contact RCMP/CSA/Child protecting agency
    Support measures
    Psycho referral
    Admit to hospital.

6. Low Birth Weight

Case 1.
45 YOF just delivered a baby weighing 2200g. Obtain a focused history.
What is your diagnosis? What supports your diagnosis in the history?
Mention 4 other factors that help you confirm your diagnosis.
What are the 2 complications this child might develop during the first 48
  hours?

Key:
Although finding the etiology is important, emphasis should focus
  on the possible complications and management.

History:
- *How old are you? What is your ethnic background? -mother*
- *Is this child full term, pre-term, post-term?*
- *Any diseases or problems during pregnancy? Infection, fever, hepatitis?*
- *Do you drink, smoke, use drugs, taking Meds?*
- *How many U/S exams performed during this pregnancy? What did the*
  doctor say?
- *Any problems with this delivery?*
- *What about your previous pregnancy?*
- *Any genetic disease runs in the family?*
- *What is your blood type? Rh? Your husband's blood group? Rh?*
- *How much weight has you gained during this pregnancy? In which part of*
  the pregnancy did you gain most of your weight?
- *Is he symmetrically small or head large, other parts small?*

History provided by the mother: Normal spontaneous delivery. U/S at 13
wk normal. No ETOH, no edema, no meds. Smoker, 2 other teenage
children normal, blood group unknown. Baby normal tone, suck,
wrinkled skin, and jaundice.

Diagnosis:
- Intrauterine growth retardation

Differential Diagnosis:
Intra-uterine growth retardation
- Hemolysis
- Placenta insufficiency
- Congenital anormally
- Premature with jaundice
- Sepsis

Complications:
1. Asphyxia-pneumonia
2. Hypoglycemia

Other: Kernicterus, lytes imbalance, anemia, hypotherma, edema, necrotizing enterocolitis, dehydration

7. Immunization

Case 1.
New immigrant mother asks about immunization for her baby. Obtain a history. How would you consult her?

History:
Which country are you from?
What vaccines has your baby had before?
Is he currently sick? Fever, meningitis, neurological disease?
Is he allergic to any vaccines? Allergic to egg white? to neomycin?
How much knowledge do you have about vaccination?
Any questions or concerns about vaccination?

Consult:
- A vaccine is a biologic product, which can elicit a specific immune response when administered to a healthy person. This immune response will protect that person from getting a specific disease.
- There are six major killers of children worldwide. They are Measles, whooping cough (petussis), tetanus toxoid, polio, tuberculosis and diphtheria. Other diseases like hepatitis, Flu and Rubella are also very bad for children's health.
- Possible adverse reactions after administering a vaccine:
  Local: induration, tenderness
  Systemic: fever, rash, prolonged crying
  Allergic: urticaria, rhinitis, anaphylaxis
- Contraindications:
  Severe illness +/- fever, allergy, immunodeficiency, unstable neurological disease
- Age 1-6:
  Initial: DPTP MMR (if >12 month) HiB
  2nd, 3rd (2 month apart) DPTP
  12 month DPTP
  4-6 Yr DPTP MMR
  14-16 Yr TdP

- Age >7:
  1st: TdP MMR
  2 months later TdP
  2 months later TdP
  every 10 years Td, No polio

- There are a total of six vaccines available clinically:
  DPTP (Diphtheria, tetanus-toxoid, Petusis-killed bacteria, Polio - inactivated virus):
- 2, 4, 6, 18 month IM
- Side effects: fever, redness, swelling
- Petussis-prolonged crying, febrile convulsion, neurology (1/100 000)
- Contraindication: anaphylaxis, current neurology disease

Hepatitis B:
- At. Birth, 1, 6 month

MMR (Measles, Mumps, Rubella – live attenuated virus):
- >12 month, 4-6 yr s/c
- Side effects: fever, Measles-like rash in 7-14 days, LN sadenopathy, arthralgia, arthritis, parotitis
- Contraindication: infants, immunocompromised, pregnancy

HiB (Conjugated to diphtheria, polysachride):
- 2, 4, 6, 18 month, no booster.
- Don't give after 7 years old

OPV (live virus):
- 2, 4, 6, 18 month oral
- Contraindication: Immunodeficient

TdP:
- Start 14-16 yrs, Q10 yrs IM
- Side effect: Anaphylaxis
- Contraindication: Immunodeficientcy

8. Cough, Asthma

Case 1.
Two year old girl complaining of cough, after being on Amoxil for 9 weeks. Obtain a history.

Case 2.
Two year old boy has been coughing for 3 weeks. He was seen by your colleague and put on amoxicillin. No response. Still coughing. Obtain a history. What are 3 possible diagnoses?

Key:
Important points on Hx for the diagnosis of asthma:
- Timing, recurrence – pattern
- trigger
- cougher/wheezer
- response to bronchodilator
- Allergy, eczema, environment, smoker, pets
- FHx

History:
- *Onset: What time does he start coughing? Did he catch a cold? Did he have a fever? Or did he contact anything?*
- *Timing: What time of the day does he likely to cough? Early morning, after exercise?*
- *Character: How does he cough? Can you describe the pattern? SOB, turing blue, wheezing?*
- *Sputum: Does he bring up any sputum? How is the sputum like? Yellow, white, sticky, or bloody, smell*
- *Is there anything that can make the cough worse? Like cold air, URTI, irritant, allergen, exercise, stress, drugs*
- *Are there clear triggers of attack?*
- *Has he ever been diagnosed asthma? being put on puffers or inhaled steroid?*
- *Has he ever been admitted to hospital for difficulty breathing?*
- *Is he a cougher or wheezer? How is the response to ventolin?*

- *Is he healthy otherwise? pulling ears? Any fever, anorexia, weight loss? Night sweats? Chest pain, hoarseness?*
- *Have you ever noticed him reflux or regurgitate food?*
- *What immunization has he had?*
- *Anybody smokes at home? Pets at home?*
- *Anybody else in the family has asthma?*

Investigations:
- CXR, CBC, PFT

Pediatric Cough Differential Diagnosis:
- Reactive airway disease, asthma
- URTI, broncheolitis, bronchitis, pneumonia-viral
- Whooping cough, vaccinations
- Foreign body, environmental smoking parents
- Cystic fibrosis
- Bronchiectesis
- TB
- Postnasal drip

Adult Cough Differential Diagnosis:
- Environmental irritant: smoking, pollutants, dusts, dry air
- LRT: Lung ca, asthma, bronchitis, emphysema, CHD, pneumonia, bronchiectasis
- URT: rhinitis, sinusitis, otitis, pharyngitis, ACE inhibitor
- Extrinsic compressive lesion. adenopathy, malignancy, aortic aneurysm
- GI: GE reflux
- Post nasal drip
- Psychogenic

Treatment:
- Treat underlying course
- Sx management:
  a. Cessation of smoking
  b. Humidification

c. Hydration

d. Encourage sputum expectorant, positional drainage,

e. Temporary cough suppression, codeine

f. Steroids and bronchiodilaters

g. Anti-acids, H2 blocker

h. ENT consult

9. Diarrhea.

Case 1.
1 year old boy, 6 months history of diarrhea. Obtain a focused history in 5 minutes.

Case 2.
2 yr diarrhea for 6 wks, Question: 3DDx, 2 Lab, 3 pertinent featured leading to Dx.

Case 3.
6 year old with diarrhea, history and differential diagnosis.

Case 4.
6 month old with 1 week diarrhea. Obtain a history in 5 minutes.

Key:
Detailed feeding history.

> 2 wks means chronic, then rule out celiac and other chronic etiology.

History:
- *What do you mean by diarrhea? How many BMs a day?*
- *What is the stool like? Watery/solid, large/small, bloody, color, smell?*
- *How did it start?*
- *Does he have a fever? Abdominal pain, vomiting -before, during or after BM?*
- *Is this child otherwise healthy? Play, sleep, growth, weight changes?*
- *Does he look pale or dry? How many times does he pee or wet diapers in the last 24 hours? Does he have tears when he cries?*
- *What does he eat? Breast-feed? Milk? How do you mix milk?*
- *Any changes in feeding pattern or formula recently?*
- *Is he stay home or being sent to day care? Any similar cases in day care? Infectious contact?*
- *Travel recently? Pets at home? eating out?*
- *Is he taking any meds? antibiotics*

• *Anybody in the family having similar problems? (Celiac disease)*

Differential Diagnosis:
With failure to thrive (FTT)
• Diet induced
• Intestinal: celiac disease, BROW barley rye oats wheat
• Milk protein allergy
• Inflammatory bowel disease
• Pancreatic: cystic fibrosis, Schwan's Syndrome
• Other: thyroid, addison's, IgA deficiency, AIDS, neoplastic

Without failure to thrive
• Toddler's diarrhea
• Infectious: bacteria, parasite, C difficile
• Lactase deficiency

Investigation:
• CBC, lytes, glucose
• Serial height, weight, growth percentile
• Stools C+S, O+P, Ovult blood, C difficile toxin, fat, pH, reducing substances
• X-ray: upper GI, barium enema
• Endoscopy, mucosal biopsy
• If FTT:
  A-1 antitrypsin, sweat chloride, thyroid function, HIV, albumen, carotene, lytes, CBC, ESR, protein

10. Attention Deficit Hyperactivity Disorder

Case 1.
Father complains that his child is hyperactive. Obtain a history and consult. What is your treatment plan?

History:
- *What do you mean by hyperactive? How is he doing in school? at home?*
- *How old is he (generally ADHD start <7yr)?*
  When did you notice the problem?
  Has anything happened at home (relationship, loss), school recently?
- *Is there any problems other than this hyperactivity?*
  Is he otherwise healthy?
  Eating, sleeping, growth, fever, night seats, weight loss?
- *Notice any changes in his Sx? Behavior?*
- *Does this type of problem run in the family?*
- *Do you think he might have access to drugs?*
- *AMPLE*
- *Antenatal, postnatal, development milestones, ear infections, delivery*

Consult:
- What he has is called attention deficit hyperactivity disorder. It usually runs in the family, however a chaotic environment can also be the cause.
- It usually starts before 7 yrs of age. Some people automatically recover before 12 yrs old, some will continue (70-80%) into adolescence or even adulthood (15-20%).

Treatment:
- Psychostimulants (Ritalin) or neuroleptics might control Sx to a certain extent, but main treatment is not pharmacological. "Cope not cure" should be the strategy both at home and at school.
- If its a grieving reaction, it will likely resolve with time. This may take up to 2 years. Talk to the teacher, understand his problem and cope with him.

11. Speech Delay

Case 1.

Parents are very worried about their 3-year-old daughter. She is slow and her speech is far behind. She only says the words "Mom" and "Dad." Her development compared with her elder brother is slow. Obtain a history. What is your differential diagnosis?

Key:

Interview parents not the child.

History:
Interview parents

- *During the interview, you will learn that it is a full term baby with no infection during pregnancy, a normal delivery and normal developmental milestones. She has Otitis media 5 times a year. They have to talk to her very loud. The examiner will ask you: Q: Diagnoses? A: Conductive deafness.*

About Mother:

- *Have you had any disease during pregnancy/breast feeding period?*
- *Did you drink, smoke, drugs, take Meds during pregnancy/breast feeding period?*
- *Any disease running in the family?*
- *Is this a full-term baby?*
- *Any difficulties/problems in giving birth?*

About child:

- *Has she had any medical issues since birth?*
- *Any fever, meningitis, ear infection, head trauma, meds?*
- *Notice any seizure activity?*
- *Is she otherwise healthy?*
- *Growth pattern when she starts sitting, walking, playing with others?*
- *What investigations/treatments she had before?*
- *What other Meds has she been taking? antibiotics?*
- *Has she ever talked?*
- *How does she communicate with others?*
- *Is she interested in communicating?*

Differential Diagnosis:

- Hearing impairment: conductive vs. neurologic, genetic, congenital infection, meningitis, Meds, otitis media
- Cognitive disability: Mental retardation, interest in communication
- Pervasive development disorder includes autism
- Selective mutism
- Landau-Kleffner Syndrome: regression of language

Case 2.

6 year old with dysphrasia, assess.
Key: Interview the child, not the parent.

Pre-assess information needed:
    Handedness
    Educational level
    Native language
    Pre-existing learning difficulty
Assess:
    Fluency, repetition
    Paraphasic error – dook for book, table for desk
    Comprehension: verbal, written
    Naming
    Writing

- *Can you hear me? Can you understand my question?*
- *Are you right handed or left handed?*
- *Observe whether the speech is fluent or not.*
- *Can you understand what people are talking about? For an example, what does it mean by: "Don't throw stones in a glass house"?* Level of comprehension
- *Can you repeat word or phrases like "No ifs, ands or buts"?*
- *Can you name objects?*

12. Failure to Thrive, Consult

Case 1.
Infant, FTT, diagnose feeding problem and consult.

Key:
Determination of Nutritional status
• Take weight/height compare to standard table
• Diet hx and GI function: appetite, N/V, C/D
• Hydration status
• Muscle bulk, subcutaneous fat
• Cheilosis, glossitis and jaundice

History:
• *How old is this baby? Is he full-term/premature?*
• *How much did he weigh at birth? How much does he weigh now (calculate)?*
• *How has he been fed? Breast/formula? How frequent?*
• *Any supplements: Fe, vitamin D, K, fluoride, Ca^{2+}*
• *Does he pause during sucking?*
• *How many BM a day? How many times does he wet his diapers daily?*
• *Has he gained any weight since birth? How much?*
• *Is he otherwise healthy and happy?*
• *Any vomiting or diarrhea? If vomit, any bile? If diarrhea, any blood?*
• *Any fever, cough, pulling ears?*
• *Does the mother have any disease? Does she drink, smoke, take Meds?*

Consult:
Breast Feed
a. Breast is the best. See obstetric and gynecology chapter.
b. Supplements: Fe 8 wks for premature, 6 months for mature
c. Mother: no smoking, drinking, drugs,
 Contraindication:
  Certain Meds: Chemo- radiation, Infection: TB, herpes

Non-breast feed

a. formula brand, should use Fe fortified, be consistent with one brand

b. 150-180 ml/kg/day

c. special formula for protein hypersensitivity, lactose intolerance, Phenylketonuria

d. whole cow's milk should not used at <9 month, because high renal protein load, poor Fe absorption, and inappropriate energy distribution

e. 2% or skim milk should not be used <12month. Fat needed for neural development

f. Vegetarian diet not recommended in first 2 year

Dietary schedule

0-4M: Breast milk, formula

4-6M: Iron enriched cereals, rice cereal first, less allergy purged vegetable, yellow-green. Not those with high nitrate: (beets, spinach, turnips)

6-9M: Purged fruits/juice, meats, fish, poultry, egg, Yorgart, no egg white

9-12M: Finger food, peeled fruit, cheese, cooked vegetable. No raw vegetables/fruits, hard, no added salts, sugar, fat, seasoning.

13. Corrosive Swallowing

Case 1.

Receive a telephone call from a mother in distress concerning her 18 month old son who has swallowed some anti-hypertensive Meds, not knowing which one.
a. Advise over telephone. b. After answering the phone, what 2 things you do?
c. List 3 initial treatments. d. What will you do differently if ingestion is corrosive?

Advice over the phone:

- *This is Dr. X at Hospital Y. Can I have your name, phone number and address please?*
- *What has he swallowed? How much (how much left in the container)? How old and how much does your child weigh?*
- *When. How long ago? After meal or before meal?*
- *Where were the meds taken? If in bathroom or cabinet, must consider multiple ingestions.*
- *Who found the baby?*
- *How is he now? Is he unconscious? Confused? Is he complaining about pain in the chest/abdomen? What Sx does he have? Has he vomited? Have you tried any emetics?*
- *I want you to calm down, the ambulance will be there shortly. In the meantime, I want you to do the following:*
  Make sure he is not in further danger – remove chemicals on the skin or pills in his mouth.
  If his mind is clear, you can give him some epicac, (if not corrosive ingestion).
  If it's corrosive ingestion, or a seizure is anticipated, or decreased LOC, no emetic, let him drink copious amount of water or milk, don't induce vomiting.
  If he vomits, clean his mouth, let him swiss his mouth with water/milk.
- *If he is unconscious:*
  Turn him over one side, lift his chin, tilt his head, make sure airway is patent, sweep the mouth

Check his skin color and breathing (10 Sec), if not breathing, do mouth to mouth 2x, check breathing again
Check his pulse at neck, if no pulse, lay him on his back, start chest compression, if <8yr, 5 compression per breath, if >8yr, 15 compression per 2x breath, then reassess
- *The ambulance is on its way, make sure to carry the poison bottle with you when the ambulance arrives*
- *If anything happens during this period, call me. I'll sit right in front of the phone.*

After answering the phone, 2 things to do:
- Contact National Poison Information Service for advise/information
- Inform ER staffs, prepare patients coming. IV line, oxygen, ipecac, antidote, charcoal ready

Initial treatments in ER:
- Stabilize, ABC, monitor vitals, IV hydration, NG, Foley
- Specific antidote
- Activated charcoal: 50-100g (adult) or 30-50g (child) through NG
- Optional: Syrup of ipecac 15-30 ml followed by large amount of fluids intake
- Blood work: toxic screen (blood and urine), CBC, PTT INR, osmolarity
- For corrosive ingestion:
  Look for signs of perforation of esophagus and stomach
  Absolutely no induction of vomit

14. Vomiting

Case 1.

A six-week-old presents with 3 days of vomiting. The nurse is weighing the baby. Obtain a history from the mom. What in the history points to the diagnosis? What lab investigations would you do? What is your diagnosis?

History:

- *When started?*
- *Relation to feeding*
- *What does he vomit out? (Vomitus)*
- *Pattern of vormit: ? Projecting*
- *Hungry afterward?*
- *BM, urine change? – dehydration*
- *Weight gain*

History **given:**

- Vomiting projectile, 15 min after feeding, still hungry, crying, won't settle, less BM and less urine
- Mom thinks he is not gaining as much weight this week. Query bile in the vomitus because it looked greenish
- No FHx of pyloric stenosis, but other kids in the family had problems with vomiting.
- No changes in feeding regime – similac

Investigations:

- Abdominal X-ray, U/S

Diagnosis:

- Pyloric Stenosis

15. Mom Finds "Pot" in Son's Laundry and Asks What She Should Do?

Key:

HEADS– Home, Education, Activity/affect/anger, Danger, Sex
PACES-Parents/peers, Accidents/alcohol/drugs; Cigarettes;
  Emotional; School/Sexual

Management:
- Work to set up initial confrontation. Getting them into treatments requires special skills.
- Present the problem as a disease, genetic, CNS basis.
- Blame partly the drug itself, it presents a serious threat to health and well being.
- Stress that once the problem is discovered, it's the responsibility of the individual to get help.
- Don't focus on the amount consumed, be ready to promise stop
- Refer to support groups.
- Involve not only the patient, but also the family .
- Emphasize risk of using IV drugs, alcohol, violence, sex

16. Epilepsy, Management

Case.
Teenager has increasing seizures, history of epilepsy. Manage.

Keys:
1. Compliance of medications
2. Alcohol/drugs as possible etiology

Management:
1. Removal of causative and precipitating factors
Rule out and treat:
- CNS infections, such as bacteria/viral meningitis
- Electrolyte disturbances such as hyponatremia, hypocalcemia
- Endocrine disturbances such as hypoparathyroidism, islet cell adenomas
- CNS neoplasms

2. Physical and mental hygiene
Inquire about:
- Loss of sleep
- Abuse of alcohol and other drugs
- Amount of exercise? Over excersise
- Psycosocial difficulties

3. The use of antilipetic drugs
Inquire and consult:
- Compliance of medications.
- Types of medication: certain drugs are more effective in a particular type of seizure.
- Initially, only one drug should be used and the dosage increased until sustained therapeutic level has been assured.
- If seizures are not controlled by the first drug, a different drug should be tried, but frequent shifting of drugs is not advisable. Each drug should be given an adequate trial before another is substituted.

- In changing medication, the dosage of the new drug should be increased gradually to an optimum level while the dosage of the old drug is gradually decreased.
- If seizures are still not controlled, a second drug can be added.
- It may help to have the patient chart daily medication as well as the number, time and circumstance of seizures.
- Monitor serum levels to ensure efficacy and watch for toxicity.
- Watch for interactions with other drugs which may cause variations in serum level.

4. Surgical elimination of epileptic foci.
Location of the discharging focus require careful analysis of clinical and EEC, etc.

17. Anemia

Case 1.
12 month male infant noted to be pale. Take a focus history in 5 minutes, diagnosis?

Key:
Confirm diagnosis, search for etiology.

History:
- *Really pale or only the mother's impression? When did you notice?*
- *Any changes over time?*
- *Any Sx: pica, dysphasia (esophageal web), cheilitis, Glossitis*
- *Is this a full term baby? Any disease or meds during pregnancy?*
- *How is he doing after birth? Gaining weigh? When did he lift his head, roll over, sit by himself?*
- *How is he fed? Fed breast or milk? Iron added, Calcium added?*
- *Any diarrhea?*
- *Is he healthy otherwise? Ever admitted to hospital for anything?*
- *Any Sx of fever, infection, liver/kidney disease*
- *FHx of anemia, ethnic background*

Diagnosis:
This Dx is common in age 3-18 months; after 18 months, must investigate blood loss (esophagitis, PUD, Meckel's IBD, Celiac disease).

Other conditions: thalassemias, sickle cells disease-present at 6-9 month with anemia, jaundice, painful crisis, splenomegaly, infections, cholelithiasis.

Chapter 5. Psychiatry and Neurology

1. Bipolar Disorder

Case 1.
Obtain a history from a patient with bipolar disorder.

Case 2.
32 YOM, one month history of special thoughts "He is God's messenger on earth, he wants to sacrifice his children." Take history in 8 minutes and in the last 2 minutes answer questions.

Key
6S: Sleep, Speak, Spending, Sex, Self-esteem, Suicide
AEA: Appetite, Energy, Activity
3 Sx last at least 1 wk

History:
- *Hi, I am Dr. X and you are . . .*
- *I understand that you have had some mood changes recently; can you tell me a little more about it?*
- *How do you actually feel? How is it affecting your life?*
  R/o secondary cause and general medical condition (GMC).
- *When did you start having mood problems?*
- *Has anything happened at home (loss, relationship), at work?*
- *Were you sick, taking any meds, using drugs, alcohol?*
- *Have you had a stroke, trauma, tumor, infection – include HIV*
- *Do you have thyroid (hyper, hypo), adrenal (Cushings) Parkinson's, or nutritional (Vit B12) disease?*
- *Major depression Sx:*
  How is your appetite? Have you lost any weight?
  Do you sleep well?
  Any changes in your mood?
  How do you think about your self? self-esteem
  Do you feel guilty at times?
  Have you ever thought of killing yourself?
  Are you able to concentrate?
  What about your energy, interest/libido?

- *Mania*

  Do you sometimes have different moods? Interview with patient's relative, if available.

  Are there times when you do something without thinking of its consequences?

  Spending, activity/consequences, sleepless, flying ideas and speedy speak, Sex, Self-esteem, suicide. Minds slow down/speed up, increased goal related activity, distraction, judgment; irritable mood

  Should ask questions mixed together.

- *SHx:*

  Who do you live with? Can you get any help from home when you run into trouble?

  What is your daily responsiboity?

- *PMHx, FHx:*

  Similar episodes in the past? Treatment/response?

  Attempted suicide before?

  Any family members with a similar disease?

Manage mania

  Plan: certify and admit

  Reason for certification: harmful to others

2. Anxiety

Case 1

26 YOM brought by wife regarding runaway/anxiety. Obtain a history and assess.

Key:

Assess severity, psychiatric and general medical conditions.

History
Assessment of severity

• *Is this something new or is it an ongoing problem?*
• *Onset, quality, intensity and duration:*
  When did you start noticing this problem?
  Did anything happen at that time? trauma, stress, GMC
  How severe? How long does this feeling last?
  Does anything make it worse/better?
• *Cause:*
  Usually under what conditions do you (he) try to run?
  Any special situations or things you are not comfortable with?
  Why are you scared of such a situation? Did something happen previously?

Assessment of psychiatric disorders

• Check for 3 subjective experiences of:
1. Motor symptoms of tension: tremor, restlessness
2. Autonomic hyperactivity: dyspnea, palpitation, sweating/cold clammy hands, dry mouth, dizziness, gastrointestinal distress, polyuria
3. Vigilance and scanning: "on edge," restless, exaggerated startle response, concentration problems, sleep problems, irritable
• *Are you scared of that situation: How do you actually feel?*
• *What Sx will you have? (STUDENTS, Fear 3 Cs)*
  Sweating: Tremor; Unsteadiness; Depersonalize; Excessive HR, Nausea/vomit; Tingling; SOB
  Fear: dyinging, loss of control, going crazy

3Cs: *chills, choking, chest pain*
• *How do you try to deal with this problem?*

Assessment of medical disorders

• *What medical issues do you currently have? What Tx? Any concerns, fears regarding this disease and Tx?*
• *Do you have thyroid disease, palpations, heart dysrhythmia?*
• *Are you taking any Meds? Recreation drugs? Alcohol?*
• *FHx: Does a similar problem run in your family?*
Childhood:
When you were a child, was there anything special you were afraid of? How come?
General anxiety disorder:
At least 6 months concerning at least 2 different issues

3. Schizophrenia

Case 1

52 YOF, 3 days posthysterectomy, complains of creeping insects, hearing music. Obtain a history, perform a MSE.

Case 2

65 YOF worried that there is radiation leaking into her house. Obtain a history and form an assessment. Do a mental status exam and give your diagnosis. 10 minutes.

Key:

Ask about drugs, alcohol and meds taken
Assess potential danger to self and/or others

History:

- *Identify date, source of Hx and reliability*
- *Do you feel unduloy anxious or depressed?*
- *Do you repeat certain tasks over and over again?*
- *Do you feel people are out to get you? against you?*
- *Do you hear or see things that are not there?*
- *Do you ever lose a sense of yourself or your environment?*
- *For Anxiety: does a particular environment provoke the symptoms?*
- *For Depression: Are there suicidal thoughts?*
- *For Schizophrenia: Have you had any auditory hallucinations?*
- *Do you believe others control your thoughts?*
    When did you start worrying about this?
    Is this thought always there? or does it go away at times?
    Have you ever had thoughts of killing others?
    Are you on a special mission?
- *How do you cope with this?*
- *Stressor, associated Sx*
- *PMH: Psychiatric disorders/treatment and hospitalization/suicide attempts*
- *AMPLE r/o GMC*
- *FHx: social support*
- *Personal Hx: perinatal, childhood, dreams, fantasies, occupation, marriage,*

relation
• *Predisposing precipitating, perpetuating and protecting factors*

Assessment: can follow previous approach
• Hx, Psychiatric Sx (Characteristic delusion, hallucination, disorganized speech, behavior, negative Sx) severity
• Last how long (at least 6 months), social/occupational dysfunction
• R/O Schizo-affective disorder, mood disorder GMC, substance abuse

Mental status exam
1. Observe patient's interaction with environment, response to doctor's self introduction
2. Body appearance, posture, body movement, gait, facial expression
   • Speech: voice tone, pace, clarify, word and sentence pattern
   • appearance, grooming/hygiene, odor
3. Mini-mental (MMSE). See Station #8.
4. Insight: How do you feel about yourself?
   • How do you cope with daily stress?
   • Identify depression, mania, anxiety and follow their direction
5. Judgment
6. Abstractive reasoning. Am I taller than you? What does it mean to not throw stones in a glass house?
7. Thought content: Do you have thoughts or feelings that you are unable to control?
   Do you have trouble making daily decisions?
8. Thought processing: tangentiality, loosening associations, word salad, neologism, echolalia
9. Coherency and relevance
10.Intelligence

Axis I. Clinial disorder
Asix II. Personality, mental retardation
Axis III. GMC
Asix IV. Psychosocial and environmental
Axis V. Global asessment of funtioning

4. Somatization/Conversion Disorder

Case 1

Old lady c/o of multiple aches and pains. She has been seen by many physicians and extensively investigated with no diagnosis. Saw your partner yesterday and not satisfied with the answers.

Case 2

Female complains of blindness, normal report from ophthalmologist. Obtain a history

Case 3

69 YOF, worried about gastric Ca-somatoform disorder.

Case 4

Elder lady, lipoma removed from axilla. Doctor discussed with the diagnosis with her but she thinks it's cancer. She is worried. Obtain a history and MSE.

Case 5

A lady complains of blurred/tunnel vision. No organic problem. Take a history.

Key

Differentiate somatization from organic disease
Define underlying psychopathology

History

1. *Timing and precipitants*

When do you start feeling this pain (not able to see things)?
Is it sudden or gradual? How does it affect your daily activity?
Has anything happened at home (loss, relationship, financial), at work?
Have any stressful events happened?
Is there anything you are worried about?

2. *Quality*

Can you describe the pain a little more for me?
OLDCARS. How severe? How frequent? How long does it last?

Does it wake you up at night?

Notice any changes?

Does any situation make it better/worse?

Associated Sx

Do you experience nausea, appetite change, or vomiting (2GI)? BM change, weight change?

Any shortness of breath? (cardiopulmonary symptoms)? Chest pain?

What about interests in sex (1 sex)? What about pain during sex?

Any sensation/movement problem (1 pseudoneurological)? numbness/weakness/tingling/paralysis?

Interest/self-esteem/mood/concentrate/period/activity/energy

4. Primary gain:

Proceeding conflicts or stress, to reduce unconscious anxiety.

Is there anything worrying you now? Is anything else bothering you?

5. Secondary gain

Who do you live with? What do they do when you get sick?

What is your job responsibility?

Does your supervisor give you less work or an easier job when you are sick?

Can you get compensation for this? Is this work related?

What will happen to you if you are not sick at this moment?

Will they cut your benefit? Is there a particular job or responsibility you have to take?

Attitude

What do you think about these pains?

Do you think they represent a serious illness?

Is it bothering you a lot?

How do you cope with it?

6. La bella indifference

What will you think if we really find some serious organic disease?

Consult

- I understand that this pain and discomfort is real, very bothersome and significantly compromises your daily activity. You are doing a very good job coping with such discomfort.

- Based on previous investigations and lab reports, there is no evidence that you are having any serious damaging organic disease, however stress can affect body system function resulting in multiple discomforts at the same time or in sequence.

- Now I have a general understanding of your story. What I am going to do next is a thorough PE and a review of your old charts.
- I'd like to see you once a week on every Wednesday afternoon. We'll deal with this together. During this time, try to relax. If anything come up in your mind, write it down and we'll discuss it next time. After reviewing your old chart, we'll discuss what to do next. We don't want to repeat anything unnecessary, but we don't want to miss anything important, as well.
- I am not going to prescribe anything at the present time which might do you harm.
- Minimize Meds: may give depression-anti-depressants, anxiety-benzodiazepine, psychotic-phenothiazine
- I'd like to refer you to a psychiatrist for consultation (pt may resist) whenever it's appropriate for you
- Any questions?

Points to Remember in Management:

- Remove Sx: reassurance, education and suggestion to reduce anxiety.
- Manage internal conflict.
- Assure the patient that Sx are self-limited, will recover gradually.
- Explain the results of medical workup without denying the patient's discomfort.
- Encourage discussing psychosocial problems and set up a regular schedule of appointments for further elaboration and supportive therapy. Make clear that he need not have a phsycial problem to see a doctor. Avoid Prn appointments.
- Treat the underlying psychological problem specifically, don't try nonspecific suppression with tranquillizers.
- Don't try to remove or cure Sx. Acknowledge the suffering and provide the support. Avoid the use of Meds and extensive work up. Make adaption chronic discomfort the goal of care.

5. Anorexia Nervosa

Case 1

16 YOF experiencing recent weight loss is concerned about anorexia nervosa. Take Hx, MSE, consult

History

- *When* *did you notice your eating problem?*
- *What do you think about your weight?*
- *How long has it been bothering you? How much do you think you should weigh?*

*Any **weight change** recently? How much did you weigh before/now? What was your maximum/minimum weight?*

- *What do you eat? How much do you eat each day? Can you remember what you have eaten in the last 24 hours?*
- *Do you skip any meals? Ask about the diet? Ask about weight loss?*
- *Ask about food binges?*
- *Do you feel fat?*
- *Do you have a fear of gaining weight?*
- *Are you preoccupied with the diet and food?*
- *Ask about sexual relationships?*
- *Ask about social life?*
- *Ask about depression (insomnia, crying)*
- *How much **exercise** do you do? What kinds of exercise do you do?*
- *What about your **period?** Have you missed any?*
- *Tell me something about your childhood? Have you ever been **abused?***
- *Some people try to vomit what they have eaten after a meal, have you ever done that? How frequently?*
  *Have you tried using **pills** to lose weight? Laxatives, diet pills, diuretics?*
- *What do you think about yourself generally?*
- *Have you ever thought about **killing yourself?** Any serious attempts?*
- *Are you suffering from any **serious disease**? Pain?*

Symtoms

- *Do you feel tired? Dizzy? Thirsty?*

- *Notice any change in you skin, hair, abdominal pain?*
- *Any rectal bleeding?*
- *How about your mentrual period in terms of regularity and amount?*
- *Whom do you live with? Is everything all right at home?*
- *Is everything OK at school? what job do you have?*
- *Do you drink/smoke/use drugs/take meds*
- *AMPLE*

MSE
- General appearance/behavior
- Speech
- Affect/mood
- Thought process: Circumstantially tangentially, flight of ideas, loosing association
- Thought content: Delusion (fixed false belief), obsession, preoccupation
- Dream content/recurrent themes, phobias, suicidal/homicidal ideation
- Perception: hallucination, illusion (misperception), depersonalization, derealization
- Cognition: orientation, memory, intellectual function (concentration, abstract)
- Judgment
- Insight
- Formulation: predisposing, precipitating, perpetuating, and protecting factors

Consult
- How tall are you? Your ideal body weight would be . . .
- Now your weight is below . . %. Appropriate body weight is very important for your health.
- Sx: Dizziness, no period for >3 months, palpation and abnormal lab findings all related to the weight loss.
- You could have a serious arrhythmia and experience sudden death. Purging also causes irreversible erosion of tooth enamel and cardiac arrhythmia.

- You certainly wouldn't want that to happen. This is a serious issue.
- Fist of all, I would like you to stop all the pills, laxatives and diuretics. You might feel a little discomfort like constipation after stopping the laxatives; another way is to gradually stop using them.
- You must keep your weight above 60% (85% according to height). If you can't do this, I'll have to admit you to the hospital for nutrition.
- You should eat more; try a family supervised diet, aiming to gain 1-2 lb/week until you reach 85% of ideal weight or until you have a normal period.

Monitor: I need you to come here once a week to measure your weight, vitals, and blood potassium to make sure you are doing OK.

- psycho referral

Hospitalize if:
a. Weight loss >40% or >30% in 3 months, or rapid progressive
b. Persistent hypokalemia unresponsive to outpatient treatment
c. Urgent: cardiac arrhythmia; syncope, severe dizziness or listless; severe depression-suicidal

6. Depression

Case 1
16 YOF feels down. Take a history.

History
1. OLDCARS
When did you start feeling this way?
Has anything happened at home (recent death, relationship, financially) at work?
Notice any changes in Sx? Does anything make it worse/ batter?
2. R/O organic cause
Do you have pain or any body discomfort at all?
Can you point out where it hurts you the most?
Are you suffering from or being treated for any disease right now?
3. Neurovegetive Sx
Do you have problems with sleep? Do you wake up very early in the morning?
Have you stopped participating in some activities?
Are you feeling sad, worthless and/ or hopeless?
Do you have trouble concentrating?
Have you lost interest? Libido
Energy: can you do half of your previous daily work?
Appetite, weight loss
Feelings of guilt
Mood change
Have you ever thought about killing yourself?
How are you going to do that? (plan)
What do you think about yourself?
Do you use drugs, drink, smoke?
Have you had any serious illness/ trauma/ admission before?
4. What Meds are you currently taking?
Do you smoke, drink, or use recreational drugs, or have you used them before at some point?
5. Psychosocial
Who do you live with? How is your family environment?

Are you financially stable?
What are your daily responsibilities?
Is there anyone who can help you when you run into trouble?

6. **PMHx, FHx**
Similar episodes before? How were they treated? Did it work?
Do any family members have a similar probem?

Differential Diagnosis
• depression, dysthymia, bipolar, schizoaffective, hypothyroidism

Hospitalize if
• Risks of homicide, suicide, inability to care for self, no family support, rapid progressing sx

7. Suicide

Case 1

16 YOF attempts suicide by ingesting ASA. She is medically cleared. You are asked to assess her to clear her psychologically.

History

- *Can you tell me why you tried to kill yourself this time?*
- *Are there problems at home (abuse, argument), school, among peers, or financially? argument with parents or between parents, loss of parent/divorce, current or threatened loss of close relationship, failing grade, loss of interest/bored*
- *Will that problem still be there when you get home?*
- *Are you going to handle the problem differently?*
- *Have you ever been diagnosed with psychiatric illness? Are you taking any Meds for that?*
- *Have you ever lost control of yourself or been controlled by outside influences?*
- *Can you hear any bizarre voices or see things that other people can't hear/see?*
- *Any mood changes recently?*
  Do you feel depressed?
  What do you think about yourself? Great, worthless, or OK
  Do you feel panic/anxiety?
  What abut sleep/appetite/weight loss/interest/concentration/energy/self-esteem?
- *Are you sick? Severe pain or discomfort somewhere?*
- *Do you drink, smoke, use drugs?*
- *Have you ever tried to kill yourself before? Are you going to try to kill yourself again?*
- *How are you going to kill yourself? What is your plan?*
- *Whom do you live with? Do you live alone?*
- *Are your family members able to help you when you have difficulty? Any family members tried to kill themselves?*

Assessment of Patient

- planned or impulsive
- lethality of atempt
- chance of discovery
- reaction to being saved
- triggers, cause and precipitants
- previous attempts
- mental status

SADPERSONS: Sex-male; Age>60; Depressed; Previous attempt; Ethanol; Rationalized Suicide in family; Organized plan; No spouse; Serious illness

Assessment of Family

- appreciation of patient's condition and risk
- ability to monitor and deal with crisis, provide of support
- other social support, peers, friends
- family psychiatric history

Contract

- *Now would you promise me, whenever you run into trouble, come and talk to me*
- Never prescribe more than a weeks supply or a total 1g of tricyclic if there is a suicidal risk.

Case 2

Sleeping pill overdose, manage

Key

Suspected overdose when: decreased level of consciousness or a young patient with life threatening arrhythmia, trauma, and bizarre presentation

Primary Survey: ABCs

Management

D1: a. ACLS

  b. Universal antidote: Oxygen
     Thiamine 100 mg IM/IV
     D50W. Glucose 50% 100 ml (1g/Kg. 50 Kg, 50g)
     Nalaxone 2 mg IV, then 0.1 mg/kg drip
D2: Draw blood
   CBS lytes, BUN, Cr, ABGs, SO2, glucose, osmality
   Drug level, drug screen if uncertain
   Ca^{2+}, Mg, PO4, albumen, ketone, LFTs, lactate
   Urine analysis
D3: Decontamination
   Ocular – irrigate
   Skin – remove clothes, wash
   GI – activated charcoal, gastric lavage, whole bowel irrigation,
   endoscopic removal, ipecac
D4: Specific antidote
   a. Expose
   b. Full vitals, ECG monitor, X-ray, etc.
• Go back, reassess, and take a secondary survey, examine
• Contact National Poison Information Centre

8. Mini-mental Status Examination

Case 1
68 YOF, post hip replacement surgery. Seeing spider on the wall, do MMSE.

Case 2
30 YOF presents with forgetting social engagements, forgetting the day of the week, but she does remember the month, the year and her age. Do an appropriate neurological exam (MMSE) in 10 minutes

Total maximum score 30
I am going to ask you a few questions. Some of them may sound silly but they help me to assess your mental status, allright?

Orientation
First I'd like to check your orientation about the time and place location

		Score
Could you name this hospital		
Name this building	1	
What floor of the building are you on?		1
What city are you in now?		1
What state/province are you in now?		1
What country are you in now?		1
Time		
What is the year?		1
What month is it?		1
What season of the year is it?		1
What day of the week is it?		1
What is the date today?		1

Registration
Now I'd like to check your memory, I am going to name 3 objects.
After I have named them, I want you to repeat them.
Remember what they are because I am going to ask you to name them again in a few minutes.

Please repeat the three items: apple, car, pencil   3

Calculation _or_ spelling – choose only 1 out of the following two questions

Calculation   5

Can you subtract 7 from 100 until you reach 65? 93, 86, 79, 72, 65

Spelling

Now I am going to spell a word forwards, and I want you to spell it backwards. The word is: World, W O R L D

Please spell it backwards

Recall

What are the 3 items I asked you to memorize?   3

Language tests

Naming

Show your wrist watch and pen to the patient, what is this called?

Watch   1

Pen   1

Repetition

I'd like you to repeat the phrase after me (only one attempt is allowed)

"No ifs, ands or buts"   1

Reading and understanding

Read the words on the page and do what it says. Hand a paper written "close your eyes" to the patient

Patient closes his/her eyes   1

Listen to instructions

I am going to give a piece of paper

When I do, take the paper in your right hand   1

fold it in half with both hands and   1

put the paper down on your lap. Give order only once   1

Writing

Please write a complete sentence   1

Sentence should have a subject and a verb, and should make sense. Spelling and grammar doesn't count.

Construction/drawing/copying ability

Please copy the drawing on the same paper   1

Patient is correct if the two 5-sided figures intersect and if all angles in the 5-sided figures are preserved.

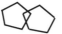

9. Cranial Nerve Examination

I:	Smell, each nostril separately
II:	Visual acuity, visual field, fundus, pupil light response
III, IV, VI:	Eye movement, near reaction, nystagmus
V:	Motor: Masseter and temporalis, open jaw with or without resistance
	Sensory: 3 branch distribution
	Reflex: Jaw jerk and corneal response
VII:	Facial expresssion: show teeth, close eye (resistance), blow
	Tighten neck muscles, hyperacusis
	Anterior 2/3 tongue, sensation, taste
VIII:	Hearing, Rinne and Weber test
IX:	Pain of tonsillar fona sensation, posterior 1/3 tongue
	Gag reflex
X:	Palatal movement and gag reflex. Say Ah----
XI:	Sternomastoid – rotate head
	Trapezius – shrug shoulder
XII:	Tongue movement and appearance

Note:

Rinne Test: Use tuning fork to compare air conduction with bone conduction.

Normal: Air conduction > bone conduction

Conductive Loss: Bone conduction > or = air conduction

Weber Test: Place tuning fork on middle of head.

Normal: Sound equally loud in both ears

Conductive Loss: Sound lateralizes to "poorer" ear

10. Seizure, Consultation and Management

Case 1

Idiopathic seizure disorder, patient asks about getting a driver's license. Hx and consultion.

Case 2

Consult a patient wishing to stop anti-convulsant therapy

Case 3

16 year old on Dilantin, previously well controlled, has had 3 seizures in the last month. Asks for better medication. Consult

Keys

- Is this episode indeed a seizure? What are the pattern and associated characteristics? Underlying cause?
- Is the Patient: (1) Under regular medical supervision, so that Dr aware of more seizure activity? (2) Truthful about frequency of seizures? (3) Compliant with Meds (4) Can seizure be prevented by the Meds taken? (5) Using alcohol or other drugs?

Hx: Take history from patient/witness

- *At what age did you start having seizures?*
- *How frequent you are having an attack? How long does the episode usually last?*
- *What was it like when you (him) were having an attack? Did you (him) get hurt, like tongue bite?*
- *Do you (him) lose conscious? Urine incontinence? Does it start from one part and then spread to other places?*
- *Do you get confused afterwards?*
- *Usually what situations would cause an episode? Sleep deprivation, drugs, ETOH. Do you know it's coming? aura?*
- *Any investigations/treatment? How well does the meds work?*
- *Are you taking drug regularly? What are you taking? Dose? Have you ever missed a dose? How frequent do you miss the medication?*
- *How long you are not having an attack?*

- *PMHx: Have you had birth injury, head trauma, meningitis, stroke before?*
- *FHx: Is there other people having similar seizure in your family?*
- *Do you drink, smoke, using drugs like insulin, bezodiazepine?*
- *What is the situation at home or at work?*

Consult about Medication

- Types of medication: Certain drugs are more effective for a particular type of seizure.
- Single therapy preferred. Initially, only one drug should be used and the dosage increased until sustained therapeutic level has been assured.
- If seizures are not controlled by the first drug, a different drug should be tried, but frequent shifting of drugs is not advisable. Each drug should be given an adequate trial before another is substituted.
- In changing medication, the dosage of the new drug should be increased gradually to an optimum level while the dosage of the old drug is gradually decreased.
- If seizures are still not controlled, a second drug can be added.
- It may help to have the patient chart daily medication as well as the number, time and circumstance of seizures.
- Monitor serum levels to ensure efficacy and watch for toxicity. Watch for interactions with other drugs which may cause variations in serum level.
- Major cause of failure to control seizures is non-compliance. Should check compliance, drug level, preciptating factor, family situation.
- Greater relapse group: complex partial seizure with generalization; abnormal EEG before/unchanged after treatment; require Valprate; Positive FHx; EEG generalized spike/wave activity.

Counsel about driver's license

a. In general, states and provinces require a seizure free interval of 6 months to 1 year before reapplication for a driver's license. Continue supervision by a physician is mandatory.

b. Spontaneous seizure, no driving until neurological exam to determine cause

c. If no epileptic activity, can drive a class 5-6 (car/motor cycle), professional drivers class 1-4 have to be seizure free without meds for at least 1 year.

d. Any type to license if (1) no meds, no seizure >5 years, (2) febrile seizure or seizure due to toxicity, (3) Seizure occur only during sleep or at waking up >5 years, plus 2 normal EEG.

e. No driving, climbing, or operating heavy machine if (1) on meds and drinking alcohol, (2) within 12 months brain surgery for seizure.

Advise: Don't drive >6 hr at a time, don't drink alcoohol, avoid stressful or fatigue situations.

Consult for stopping Meds

What was the seizure pattern when you had an attack?
What was the EEG pattern?
What is the EEG show after Meds?
Have you ever required Valprate?
Any family member had seizure?
How long were you attack free?

Isolated convulsion don't warrant long-term Meds. Short-term course may be used in setting alcohol/drug withdraw.

D/C meds require at least 1-year seizure free. Child onset, primary generalized type 50% cease at age 20.

If there is no obvious self-limited etiology, usually needs long-term prophylaxis

Manage a patient with seizure status

a. ABC, 02, Cardiac, monitor

b. D50W 100 ml bolus, thiamine 100 mg/M

c. Lorazepan IV 2-4 mg

d. Draw metablock and drug screen, anti-convulsant level

e. IV phenytoin 15-18 mg loading in 250 ml NS over 20 minutes with maintenance started 12 hrs later, if not work, Phenobarbital 10-15 mg

f. Call anesthetics for indications of general anesthesia, Consider transfer to ICU

Investigate:

Draw metabolic and drug screen, anti-convulsant level

CXR, EEG, CT, MRI – if first seizure or if focal neurologic deficit elicited.

Lytes, glucose, BUN, Cr

Manage a patient with Seizure

Psychosocial

a. Educate patient and family, advise about swimming, boating, locked bathroom, operation heavy machinery, climbing heights, chewing gum

b. Pregnancy issues, counselling and monitoring blood levels closely, teratogenicity of Meds

c. Inform the prohibition to drive and requirement to notify government

d. Support groups, epilespsy association

e. F/U visits to ensure compliance evaluate changes in Sx

Pharmacological

a. Begin one major drug with a simple dosage schedule, adjust dose to achieve low therapeutic range

b. If not controlled, maximize safe dose, if no control, change or add second drug

11. Alcoholic Neurologic Exam

Case
35 YOM just had a convulsion, Hx of alcoholism. Perform neurological Exam

Key
Eye, walk, memory, talk

Clinical presentation for alcoholics
• General: malnutrition, liver cirrhosis sign
• Acute intoxication
  Slurred speech, CNS depression, disinhibited behavior, poor coordination
  Nystagmous, diplopia, Dysarthria, ataxia, progress to coma
  Blackouts
  Risk of subdural hematoma from falls
  Frank hypotension (peripheral vasodilatation)
• Obtundation
  Associated head trauma, depressant/street drugs, hypoglycermia, hepatic encephlopathy
• Wernick'es: acute, reversible
  Ocular Nystagmous, 6th nerve palsy, gaze palsy
  Ataxia
  Vestibular dysfunction vertigo, imbalance, delirium
• Karsakoff's chronic, only 20% recover
  Marked short-term memory loss
  Difficulty in learning new information
  Anterograde amnesia
  Confabulations – elaborate, fanciful
• Withdraw
a. Mild: 6-8 hrs after intake, generalized tremor, anxiety and agitation, autonomic hyperactivity, insomnia, nausea, vomiting
b. Alcoholic hallucination: 24-36 hrs after intake, visual and auditory
c. Withdraw seizure, brief, generalized tonic-clonic

d. Delirium tremens: 3-5 days after stop drinking, severe confusion, agitation, insomnia, hallucination/delusion, tremor, tachycardia, hyperpyrexia, diaphoresis

PE

Inspect

General appearance: LOC, malnutrition, cheilitis, parotitis, diaphoresis

Walk-ataxia gait, imbalance

Vitals – hyperpyrexia, tachycardia

Talk

Orientation: ask and talk – confusion, obtundation, dysarthria, slurred

Self-esteem and career – confabulation, depression

Test memory – amnesia

See or hear anything strange – hallucination

Test

Nose-finger-tremor

See an object – diplopia

Eye movement-6th nerve, nystagmous

12. Cerebella Dysfunction, Ataxia, Neurologic Exam

Case
60 YOM with difficulty walking (cerebella dysfunction). Do a focused PE

Key
Changes in rate, range, rhythm and force of movement, no motor, sensory loss

PE
- General appearance: LOC, talk, attitude, facial expression, vitals
- Gait and posture: Walk balance, position, strength, wide based, ataxia, titubating posture
  Does the patient limp (trip)?
  Is one shoe worn out more readily than the other?
  Does patient stagger to one particular side?
  Does patient, despite apparently severe ataxia, seldom sustain injury?
- Eyes: Nystagmous – fast components of beats toward lesion side
- Speech: Dysarthria – scanning speech, staccato speech
- Unintentional movement: Dysdiadochokinesia repeat alternating movement
- Intentional movement
  Dysmetria – finger-nose test, gross incoordination, heel-shin
  Intention tremor – write, point to a spot
- Muscle hypotonia: Impaired check/rebound and pendular reflex
- Romberg test

DDX
- Is the weakness due to nerve or due to muscle disease?
  Nerve: sensation loss, reflex start peripheral
  Muscle: normal sensation and reflux
  Electromyogram, nerve conduction study

- Is the lesion upper motor neuron or lower motor neuron?
  UMN: increased muscle tone, spasticity, hyperreflexia, positive Babinski's sign
  LMN: flaccidity, hyporeflexia, and fasciculation, atrophy
- Is the nerve dysfunction confined to one root or dermatome or to one peripheral nerve?
  Yes: compressive neuropathy
  No: diffuse neuropathy, diabetes, alcohol excess, toxin, drug, genetic (Charcot-Marietooth)

13. Parkinson's Disease, PE

Case
60 YOM Parkinson's disease. Do focus PE

Tremor
• *Is it mainly present at rest, when you hold the hands out, or when you use your hand?*
• *Can it be relieved by alcohol?*
• *Does anybody in your family have a tremor?*

Key
TRAP: tremor, rigidity, akinesia, posture instability

PE
Vitals: – look for orthostatic change (Shy-Dragers' syndrome)
Appearance: inspect for:
    Mask like face, lack of blinking
    Blepharoclonus: fluttering of closed eyelids
    Tremor: rest, pill rolling, 4-7 HZ
    Drooling: dysphasia and tongue protrusion
Talk: Dementia (subcortical), hypophonia
Ask to:
    Close eyes: blepharocionus
    Stand: posture instability
    Walk: start hesitation, small shuffling steps, and loss of arm swing, first step retardation, festinating, propulsion, stoop
    Move arm: rigidity (lead pipe/cogwheel), akinesia, and bradykinesia

14. Meningitis

Case 1

a. *18 YOM, fever, vomiting, headache, and drowsiness for 2 days, recent URTI. Do PE*

b. *GCS 8, meningeal irritation (+), no focal finding, DDx*

c. *Investigations*

Case 2

Examine a 45 YOM with meningitis. He has upgoing plantars bilaterally. He had a convulsion complicating his meningitis, PE

Case 3

65 YOF, one wk hx of flu-like symptom, T 38.5 C, seizure for the 1st time in her life. Do PE in 8 minutes.

PE: −confusion −neck rigidity −straight leg raising-limited −fundus exam

Q: Dx? 1. Mengitis, 2. Elevated ICP

Keys

Signs leading to Dx include:

Fever, Rash (meningococcus)

Meningismus, neck rigidity, Bruzinski and Kerning sign

Altered mental status, confusion

Other: irritability, photosensitivity, vomiting

PE

- ABC and vitals
- General appearance, toxic, signs of sepsis
  Petechial rash
  Signs of pneumonia and endocarditis
- Cranial nerve, pupil, HEENT
- Entire nervous system, paralysis, sensation, movement, reflex, pathological reflex, lateralizing sign
- 5N's: neck, noggin, needle, ENT, neurology
- LOC Glasgow coma scale

Eye	Extremity	Speech
4 Open spontaneously	6 To command	5 Communicating well
3 To speech	5 point to pain	4 confused conversation
2 To pain	4 Withdraw from pain	3 inappropriate words
1 No response	3 decorticate, flex	2 incomprehensible
	2 Decerebrate, extension	sounds
	1 paralysis	1 no speaking at all

- Meningeal Signs
  Kernings: flexing the hip of a supine patient and then detecting the resistance or pain when the leg is extended
  Brudzinski's: flexing the neck and watching for simultaneous flexion of the hip
  Opisthotonos: hyperextension of the back with arching
- Likely bacteria:
  Infants-E. coli   2-6 yr H. influenzie
  Young-N meningococcus   >25-S. pneumonae

Investigation
a. CBC, lytes, C+S, ESR drug and toxic screen
b. Lumbar puncture: CSF pressure, cells, protein all up but glucose down means bacteria
c. X-ray CXR, sinus, mastoid
d. CT, MRI, EEG

DDx
Meningitis, Subrachnoid hemorrhage, encephalitis, trauma, ETOH/drug intoxication

15. Coma

Case 1
A 60 YOF, in coma in ER, manage

Case 2
70 YOM coma patient, perform neurologic exam

Primary survey
1. ABC
2. Resuscitation
- IV access
- Rapid blood sugar-finger prick
- Glucose, CBC. lytes, BUN, Cr, LFT and serum osmolality
- ECG
- ABG
- Give: Thiamine 100 mg IM before glucose
  Glucose 50% 50 ml if glucose <4 mmol or rapid measurement not available
  Nalaxone 0.4-2mg IV if narcotic toxidrome present
- Urine and serum drug and toxicity screen

Secondary survey
- Hx: from family, friends, police, etc.
  Acute or insidious onset
  Trauma or seizure activity
  Hx of diabetes, depression, cardiac vascular disease, TIA
  Meds, alcohol or drugs
  AMPLE
- **PE: vitals and 5 Ns**
  Racoon eyes, battle's sign
  Neck – C spine, neurogenic shock, nuchial rigidity
  ENt-otorrhea, rhinorrhea, tongue biting, breath odor, tympanum
  Needles-track marks

Neurological
  GCS
  Pupils-reactivity and symmetry
  Respiration rate and rhythm
  Apneustic or ataxic (brain-stem), Cheyne-Strokes
  (Cortical)
  Occulocephalic reflex (after C-spine clear)-dolls eye
  Oculocaloric reflex after r/o typanic membrane
  perforation, if unresponsive indicates dysfunction at low
  levels of brain stem
  Muscle tone, reflexes
  Squeeze nail bed, archilles tendon
• X-ray and CT MRI as necessary
• Re-examine frequently very important

Definitive treatment

Consult neurosurgery, neurology

16. Dementia

Case 1
55 YOF with decreased memory and increased confusion, perform neurology exam, not MSE

Case 2
Daughter of 78 YOF is concerned about mother who is withdrawn and confused. On multiple Meds. Husband died 6 months ago. Discuss with her mother's problems and management.
(Theophyllin level too high, causes drowsiness, hold, Ativan D/C, erythromycin - if no infection, D/C)

Keys
Differentiate dementia from encephlopathy
Address relative but keep eye contact with the patient

Hx
- *Has there been a change in your mood?*
- *Has your memory deteriorated?*
- *Do you have difficulty finding the right word in conversation?*
- *Have you ever become lost while travelling a familiar route?*
- *Do you have difficulty dressing?*
- *When and how did this start?*
Gradual – depression, Alzheimer's dementia
Acute – depression, delirium, infection, trauma, stroke
- *Which happened first? Memory, gait, change in mood, trauma/fall, or focal neurologic sign?*
- *How has the problem changed? Is it getting better or worse?* – rate of cognitive decline
Stepwise-multi-infarct
Slowly progressive- Alzheimer's, subacute (CJD, endocrinopathy)
- *Can she take care herself, to what degree?* – degree of social function impairment
- *How much and what does she eat? Drinking any alcohol?* – nutritional status

- *How is her mood?* – signs of depression
- *Does she feel cold all the time? any leg edema?*– hypothyroidism
- *Drug Hx: What medications has she been taking? Does she drink alcohol?* – drug toxicity
- *FHx: Any family member has similar problem?* – Dementia, depression, heart, stroke

  What are associated Sx?

  Ataxia, urinary incontinence – NPH

  Constipation, rough skin/hair, sluggish hypothroidism

  Shuffling gait – Parkinson's

  Focal neurodeficiencies – TIA
- *PMHx: Is she healthy otherwise? Any other disease?*

  HTN, DM, heart disease, hypothroidism, anemia, TIA/stroke, depression, chronic falls, syphilis, HIV, etc.
- *Hx: Where does she live? Who are her supports? Is homecare arranged?*

PE
- MSE, This is usually what they are asking for
- Look for signs of pseudo-dementia, depression, hypothroidism
- Look for signs of degenerative process, hypothyroidism, syphilis, B12 deficiency
- Focal neurological signs
- Involuntrary movement
- Pseudobulbar sign (sudden cry or laugh with least provocation), primitive reflex

17. Dysphasia

Case
68 YOM with dysphasia, assess

Key
May need help from the third party

Pre-assess information needed
    Handedness
    Educational level
    Native language
    Pre-existing learning difficulty
Assess
    Fluency, repetition
    Paraphrasic error: e.g., dook for book, table for desk
    Comprehension: verbal, written
    Naming
    Writing

- *Can you hear me? hearing difficulty*
- *Can you understand my question?*
- *Can you understand what people are talking about?*
- *What does it mean by: Don't throw stones in a glass house? – level of comprehension*
- *Are you right handed or left handed?*
- *Can you repeat word or phrases like "No ifs, ands or buts?" speech fluency*
- *Can you name objects? What is that?*

18. Post-op Hallucination

Case

52 YOF 4 days post-op hysterectomy presented with auditory and visual hallucinations. She was given Tylenol #3 and Ativan 1 mg post-op night. Take a focused history.

Key

Hx focus on key differential diagnosis

- <u>*ETOH withdrawal/Delirium tremens*</u>
Do you feel heart palpitation? Heart rate?
Is your hand shaking at times? Tremor?
Do you feel agitated or angry?
Do you sweat (diaphoresis)/
Do you drink alcohol, how much? How frequent?
- <u>*Encephalitis/meningitis*</u>
What kind of anesthesia have you had?
Is it epidural?
Any discomfort at the needle site?
- <u>*Narcotic withdrawal*</u>
Were you on any drugs?
How long have you not taken them?
- <u>*Sepsis*</u>
How high is your temperature?
What does your blood work (CBC) look like?
Do you have wound infection source anywhere?
Any other infectious disease? – Cellulitis, abscess, pneumonia, UTI, etc.
- <u>Preexisting psychotic disorder</u>
Have you had similar symptoms before?
Were you on any medication for that?
Have you stopped those medications?
- <u>Pos-op psychosis – diagnosis of exclusion</u>
Do you have any concerns about the surgery?

19. Neurology Assessment

Case: Perform neurology assessment on a patient with a neck injury.

1. Motor Exam
• Appearance bulk, tone, power
• DTR, abdominal and plantar response
• Involuntary movement: tremor, tics, myoclonus, chorea, hemiballism, fasciculation

2. Sensory Exam
• Pain, temperature, light touch
• Proprioception, pseudoathetosis, Romberg, joint position
• Vibration
• Cortical sensory function, sensory suppression
• Reflex

3. A-Z Neurologic Exam
1-vital, 2-pupil, 3-lateralize sign, 4-cranial nerve, 5-hold out stretched hand, 6-rombert, 7-gait, 8-reflex, 9-finger-nose, 10-dysdiodochoakinesia

Chapter 6. Surgery

1. Sexual Transmitted Disease, Male

Case 1.
Gay male complains of penile discharge but doesn't believe in condom use.
Obtain a history. What is the etiology and describe your investigation.

Case 2.
28 years old heterosexual male with three day history of urethral discharge.
Take a history. Give three differential diagnoses and advice.

Key
Reiter's Syndrome: Conjunctivitis + arthritis + urethritis
Be sure to include joint and eyes.

History:
STD exposure
- *How long you have you had this problem?*
- *How many partners do you have? How many partners over the past 6 months?*
- *Recent unprotected sex? Do you use condoms during sex?*
- *How long ago might you have had such a contact? (incubation)?*
- *Does your partner complain of vaginal discharge? Rectal discharge?*
Symptoms
- *Do you have any pain?*
- *Do you have an itching sensation in your penis?*
- *What color/odor is your discharge? How much discharge?*
- *Do you have any swelling or pain in your bones or joints?*
- *Do you have a burning sensation in your eyes or gritty, red eyes?*
- *Do you have a burning sensation when you want to urinate? Onset of urination or middle of it? Maybe at the end of it?*
- *Did you use the washroom in these past few days frequently?*
- *Do you have any changes in your bowel habit?*
- *Do you have anal-rectal pain, bleeding, and diarrhea, mouth pain, sore throat?*
- *Do you have fever, adenopathy, weight loss?*

- *Do you have skin rash, ulcer penile warts, ulcer, or herpes?*

PMHx

- *Is this the first time you have had this kind of problem?*
- *Have you ever had the same problem before?*
- *Have you been taking any medications or change in your medications?*
- *Do you have any other sexual transmitted disease? Or are you under any treatment for it?*
- *Do you drink alcohol, smoke, use drugs?*
- *Have you ever been diagnosed with hepatitis, TB, or other diseases?*

Physical Examination:

Pay special attention to an examination of the genitalia. Examine the penis and around the anus for wounds, ulcers, warts and discharge; examine the inguinal region for lymphadenopathy and then take the wet mount and other specimens for culture.

Etiology:

- Gonorrhea
- Chlamydia
- Trichomonas
- E. coli

Investigation:

- CBC, C+S
- Urine analysis and urine culture
- Discharge: Gram stain, Saline wet mount, KOH wet mount
- Investigation for other STDs: HbsAg, HbeAg, HIV, VDRL, CMV, HBCAg.

Consult

- Safe sex, use condoms
- HIV testing
- Investigation and treat partner
- Educate how diseases are transmitted
- No sex until complete treatment

2. Impotence

Case 1.

30 YOM complains of erectile dysfunction. He is in a new relationship with a female who is very successful in business. He is in love. No previous serious relationship. Explore cause/possible investigation.

Psychosexual History:

- *You are having difficulties with sexual function, is that right?*
- *What is the problem: desire, erection or maintaining erection?*
- *How long has it been like this? Has it started with the current relationship?*
- *Are you able to develop satisfying emotional relationships?*
- *Do you have a satisfying physical relationship?*
- *Are you heterosexual, homosexual or ambivalent?*
- *Do you use contraception? And if so, what form?*
- *Do you have problem achieving sexual arousal?*
- *Do you experience orgasm?*
- *How were your previous experiences with other women?*
- *Have you ever had a good erection/ejaculation ever since?*
- *How is your current relationship?*
- *Do you worry a lot about the possible failure every time you attempt sexual intercourse?*
- *Is that because you love her so much?*
- *Is it always not good or sometimes better? What situation usually makes it better/worse?*
- *Some people have premature ejaculation, do you have?*
- *Some people can stimulate their penis to achieve erection, can you do that?*
- *Have you ever awakened in the morning and found your penis erect?*

Secondary Cause

- *Are you suffering from any serious illness like diabetes, HTN?*
- *Any trauma or surgery in the perineal region? Spinal injury? Prostatectomy? Colorectal operation? Radiation, aortoiliac artery disease (Atherosclerosis)?*
- *Do you drink, smoke, taking any Meds, using drugs? AMPLE, FHx*
- *Notice any changes in body hair, fat distribution, or voice?*

Investigation:
- Blood: testosterone, FSH, LH, prolactin, glucose, cholesterol.
- Nocturnal penile tumescence monitor
- Doppler, penile-brachial index <0.6 suggest vascular disease
- Angiography, cavernography, penile injection
- Sacral nerve reflex latency time

Differential Diagnosis:
Psychological causes 50%:
- Young age, intermittent, no risk factor, and nocturnal penile tumescence present, able self stimulate

Organic or non psychological causes 50%:
- >50yr, constant, nocturnal tumescence absent

Risk factors:
- Endocrine: Diabetes, gonadal dysfunction, pituitary dysfunction
- Cardiovascular: HTN, atherosclerosis
- Neurologic: Problems in sacral plexus, problem in spinal cord
- Iatrogenic-anti-HTN; radiation, surgery
- Penile-postpriapism, peyronie's

3. Prostrate Cancer

Case 1.

60 YOM complains of urinary retention for 12 hrs. In/out catheterization produces 120 ml urine. Obtain a history. What is your differential diagnosis, investigation, and management.

Keys: Must ask about back pain because:
1. Vertebrae are the most common site of metastasis for prostate carcinoma
2. Back surgery/trauma can cause neurological consequences.

History:
- *Is this urinary retention a new problem for you or is it an ongoing problem?*
- *How long have you had this problem? Any changes with time?*
- *Ever notice any blood in the urine?*
- *Is it getting worse/better? Usually what situation makes it worse? What about alcohol, spicy food?*
- *Do you have problems controlling your urine? Any burning, pain while urination?*
- *How frequent do you have to go to the bathroom?*
- *Do you have belly pain, fever, cough, lower backache, weight loss?*
- *What about appetite and energy?*
- *Ever notice leg, face swelling?*
- *Any back pain or back surgery before? Spinal trauma?*
- *PMHx: AMPLE, FHx, SHx sexual*

Investigation:
- **DRE,**
- **PSA, PAP**
- **TRUS + biopsy**
- Urine analysis
- Lymph angiogram
- Bone scans
- CT

Differential Diagnosis:

- Prostate Ca
- BPH
- Cauda equine Syndrome
- Urethra obstruction (valve, stricture)

Management:

- Ca: Stage T1, 2-Radical surgery, Stage T3, 4 staging adenectomy + radiation + hormone treatment (orchiectomy, LH - RH agonist Leupromide)
- BPH:
a. Conservative management
b. Medical: Alfa-adrenergic antagonist terazosin reduce Prostate smooth muscle tone, 5-a reductase-reduce Prostate size
c. Surgery: TURP, open prostectomy, other stents, microwave, laser therapy, etc.

4. Breast Disease

Case 1.
Needs to learn how to do a self-breast exam:

How old are you? Are there any special concerns about your breast you would like to address before I start to teach you?

Timing:
• Breast self-exam should be done monthly after age 20 at 2-3 days after period ends. If no longer menstruating (menopause), pick a day e.g.: the 1st day of each month. Physician exam should be done every 1-2 years before age 40, and yearly after.

Positions:
• Sit: arm down, raise arm to behind head, then arm against hips or clench hands to each other.
• Lie: raise arm behind head, put pillow behind exam side of the chest.

Inspection:
• Size, symmetry, contour,
Nipple and areola:
• Shape, position, color, symmetry, smoothness, local retraction
Skin:
• Color, texture, venous pattern, ulceration, dimpling (orange skin), swelling
Palpation:
• Around the clock, versus quadrant exam. Look for changes in texture, symmetry, tenderness, mass (mobility, size)
• Don't forget the tail of Spence and areola for lumps or nodules
• Gently squeeze the nipple and look for discharge
Lymph Node:
• Axillary: apical, medial-lateral, anterior, posterior, sub-super clavicular LNs, contralateral nodes

Case 2.

Patient's mother and two sisters have had breast cancer. Provide a consultation.

Consult:

She will ask you:
- *Does it have any relation to food? fat, alcohol*
- *How often should I do a breast self-exam? After end of each period.*
- *What factors increase the chance of breast Ca? FHx: Previous Breast Ca, early menarche, late menopause.*
- *Do I need any other investigations? Mammogram*

You will ask her:
- *Have you ever had an operation on your breasts?*
- *Have you had any radiation to your breasts or your axilla?*
- *Do you notice anything abnormal in your breast or are you just worried about the chances of getting Ca?*
- *Tell me more about the breast carcinoma of your mother (or sister)? How old was she when diagnosed with breast carcinoma? Was it bilateral?*

You will tell her:
 If they get Ca pre-menopausal, bilateral, your chance of getting breast Ca is 5 times higher than normal population.

You will tell her:
Risk factors of getting breast Ca:
1. There are some factors we can't modify, such as:
- Genetic
- Sex
- Menarche <12 menopause >55
- Prior Hx of breast Ca
2. However, there are some factors we can change:
- Alcohol
- Smoke
- Obesity
- BCP/estrogen replacement

- Nuliparity
- Late-pregnancy
- Irradiation
- Early discovery and appropriate management is the key to a cure, if Ca:

Localized to breast - 80% 5 year survival

Localized to breast + receptor positive - 90% 5 year survival

With positive LN - 50% 5 year survival, 25% 10 year survival

- You will tell her: In order to monitor and make early diagnosis, you should:

Breast exam:

1. Self examination:
- monthly after age 20,
2. By physician:
- 1-2 times before 40,
- Yearly after age 40

You will tell her:

Indications for Mammogram:

Canadian task force on preventive health care:

A1: Screening: every 1-2 year for women ages 50-69 years.

A2: Women ages 40-49 years with above average risk of developing breast Ca.

B: Nipple discharge without palpable mass.

C: Metastatic adenocarcinoma of unknown origin.

Case 3.

60 YOF complains of nipple discharge. Her mammogram shows microcalcification. Take a history and provide a consult.

History:

- *When did you start noticing discharge?*
- *What color is it? Bloody, yellow, green, white? How much? Smell?*
- *Is it from both sides or just one side?*
- *From one spot or multiple spots?*

- *Is it spontaneous, intermittent or persistent? Is it produced by pressure at a specific spot or all over?*
- *Notice any change related to menstral period?*
- *Is there any pain?*
- *Are you otherwise healthy? Do you have fever, cough? Bone pain? Weight loss?*
- *Did you have breast Ca before?*
- *Any family members had breast Ca?*
- *Notice any changes in the skin, mass in that breast or mass in the axillary?*
- *Do you remember at what age you started to have a period? When it stopped?*
- *How many pregnancies? How many children? Were they breast fed?*
- *Do you smoke? Drink? Using drugs? Taking Meds, particularly estrogen?*

Consult:

- Nipple discharge can be associated with fibrocystic change, intraductal papilloma, or hormonal influences.
- Microcalcification can be associated with benign breast disease such as fibrocystic change, ductal carcinoma in situ or invasive carcinoma.
- A mammotome biopsy of the calcification area is essential to r/o carcinoma.
- For bloody nipple discharge, needle localized excisional biopsy can have both diagnostic and therapeutic value.
- Further investigation for metastasis include CXR, bone scan, etc.
- Prognosis determined by stage, size, local invasion, LN, distant metastasis and Estrogen receptor, etc.

Case 4.
60 YOF with a breast lump. Obtain a history.

History:
- *When did you find the lump? Do you do regular breast exams?*
- *Notice any changes in size, mobility?*
- *Any discharge, nodes in axilla, skin tethering?*

- *Any family member – Family hx of breast Ca?*
- *Age at menarche, at menopause, HRT*
- *Age at first pregnancy*
- *Previous benign breast diseases, trauma, biopsy*
- *Other breast disease: Ca, fibrocystic*
- *Other GU disease: ovarian/endometrial Ca*
- *Do you drink alcohol, smoke?*
- *Previous breast low-dose irradiation?*

Consult:

Ca risk

Painless lump – 66%

Painful lump – 11%

Nipple discharge – 9%

Local edema – 4%

Nipple retraction – 3%

Nipple crusting – 2%

Miscellaneous – 5%

- Common causes of breast lump:

<35 YO: fibrocystic, fibroadenoma, bacterial mastitis, Ca
   (uncommon), fat necrosis-rare

35-50 YO: fibrocystic, Ca, fibroadenoma, mastitis, fat necrosis

>50 YO: Ca, fibrocystic, fat necrosis, mastitis

Investigation:

- Mammogram
- Biopsy

5. Carpal Tunnel Syndrome

Case 1.

History suggests CTS. Do a focused physical exam, investigation and management.

Keys:

1. Risk factors include: Job-related repeated mild movements and trauma, pregnancy, acromegaly, myxedema, diabetes, inflammatory arthritis
2. Always examine joints above and below.

Neck, shoulder, elbows, arm, especially neck:

- pain, tenderness, point tenderness in specific parts of neck or shoulder.

Forearm and wrist

- Inspection: size of forearm, deformity
- Percussion: tender point, snuff box, crepitus
- ROM: F-E, radial-ulner deviation
- Muscle: Flexor-flexor carpi radialis/ulnariss, flexor digitorium sublimis/profundus, Extensor carpi radialis longus/ulnaris, extensor digitorium, extensor polices longus

Hand

- Inspection: deformity, skin, nails, tendon thickening, muscle wasting, and fasciculation
- Percussion: every bone/joint for swelling, tenderness, and nodules-Heberden at DIP, Bouchard at PIP
- ROM: Finger-Flexion/extension (F-E), Adduction-Abduction Thumb-F-E, add-opposition
- Muscle: Ulner nerve-1st digital interossous, adductor polices, abductor digital minimi
- Median Nerve – Thenar eminence: abductor pollices brevis, opponent pollices

Positive signs of CTS
1. Numbness: thumb, index and long fingers and radial side of ring finger
2. Thenar (base of thumb) muscle atrophy and finger weakness
3. Phelan's test: have the palmar flex for 1 minute
4. Tinel's test: tap the median nerve
5. Temperature and pulse

Investigation:
1. Nerve conduction study (NCV; nerve conduction velocity)
2. EMG (electro myelography)
3. Other: x-ray C-spine, wrist

Management:
1. Weight loss, lasix. Etiology management
2. Rest night splint
3. NSAID
4. Steroid
5. Surgery: refractory pain (>3 month), sensory loss, and muscle atrophy (doing operation, depends on results of EMG and NCV.)

3 Differential Diagnoses:
• C-spine, thoracic outlet Syndrome
• Nerve entrapment syndrome
• Arthritis
• Tendonitis

6. Abdominal Pain
Case 1.
Female, acute LLQ pain. Do a physical exam. What are three differential diagnoses and what is your investigation?

Case 2.
20 YOF complains of right flank pain. Perform a physical exam.

Case 3.
RUQ pain. Take a history. X-ray suggests small bowel obstruction, manage.

History: Abdominal Pain
- *OLDCARS*
- *When does it start?*
- *Have you had similar pain before?*
- *Is it related to BMs?*
- *Does it have radiation to anywhere?*
- *Is the pain constant or intermittent? (Colicky pain?)*
- *Does the pain wake you up at night?*
- *Did you lose any weight?*
- *Have you taken any drugs that might hurt your stomach: like aspirin, ibuprofen, steroids?*
- *Has there been a change in bowel habits?*
- *Is this pain localized/generalized, sudden/gradual?*
- *Can you show me where your pain comes from?*
- *Relation to meals, breathing, N/V, (how vomits like), diarrhea?*
- *Prior abdominal surgery, previous episodes of obstruction?*
- *Known gall bladder/kidney stones?*
- *GI: Presence and nature of vomitus, Flatus*
- *GI: appetite, time of last bowel movement, diarrhea, constipation, and effects of BM on pain*
- *GU: STD, Fever, and urine frequency*
- *Gynecology: LMP, vaginal discharge, dysparunia, and irregular menses*
- *Sexual hx: type of contraception (pill, condom), number of partners and their medical condition. Vaginal discharge, pain on intercourse*
- *Psycho: fears, concerns and expectations*

- *AMPLE*
- *PMHx: surgery, trauma, alcohol-drinking, CAD, anticoagulant therapy*
- *SHx: home, parents, siblings, smoke, drink, drugs*
- *School: attendance, performance, achievement, personal goals.*

Physical Exam: Abdominal
General appearance:
1. LOC, ABC, vitals, position
2. Dehydration, jaundice, anemia and nutrition
3. Cyanosis, cardiovascular distress
4. Does pt look septic?
5. Liver cirrhosis signs – spider nevi, etc
6. Peripheral edema
7. Leukonychia, koilonychia
Chest:
- Splinting, pleural friction rub, consolidation, chest wall
- Heart murmur, enlargement and Sx of failure
- Lung crackles

Abdomen
Inspection:
- Peristalsis
- Scar and striae
- Hernia, umbilical, inguinal
- Shape and symmetry
- Distension, make abdomen big or small
- Cullen's sign: (peri-umbilical blue discoloration due to Retropertoneal hemorrhage)
- Grey turner sign: (flank blue discoloration due to Retroperitoneal hemorrhage)
Palpation:
- light palpation for pain, deep palpation for mass
- liver, spleen kidney, ureter, bladder, aorta
- bruit pulsating mass – AAA
- Peritoneal signs: Murphy's, Rovsing`s, Psoas; Obturator, shake tenderness, cough tenderness

- Kehrs (left shoulder pain due to splenic rupture); Blumberg (rebound),Courvoisier (pancreatic cancer)
- Murphy's sign: inspiratory arrest on deep palpation of RUQ due to cholecystitis

Percussion:
- Liver-margin, spleen-9th intercostal space (traub's space)
- CVA tenderness
- Ascites-shifting dullness/percussion dullness/percussion wave
- Suprapubic dullness

Auscultation:
- BS
- Aorta and renal bruits
- Hepatic + splenic rub

Inguinal:
- Look for hernia,
- Inspection and palpatron of testicles

DRE and PV:
- Rectal mucosa, prostate, uterus.

Differential Diagnosis for case 1:
1. diverticulitis
2. Ureter stone (renal colick)
3. Ectopic pregnancy
4. PID
5. Torsion of ovarian cyst
6. appendicitis
7. Mittleschmertz
8. Irritable bowel syndrome

Investigations for case 1:
1. CBC + differential
2. Abdominal series, CXR
3. Pregnancy test HCG
4. Paracentesis, peritoneal lavage
5. U/S
6. Blood: lytes, BUN, Cr, Amylase, Bilirubin, LFTs, C+S
7. Urine/Stool analysis, C+S

8. Barium enema/upper GI, endoscopy, IVP, CT, ERCP

Physical Exam for case 2:

- Observe patient undressing shirt, spine alignment, ROM, swelling, muscle spasm, CVA.
- Observe leg movement, walk, and gesture
- Palpate CVA tenderness, suprapubic tenderness
- GU, DRE

Management for case 3:

- Admit
- NG, Foley
- IV, correct lytes and acid-base
- Conservative: laxative, enema, rectal tube
- Surgery

For Flank pain:

Differential Diagnosis:

- Kidney stone, renal infarction, pyelonephritis, spinal or par spinal muscle spasm
- Indication of renal stone: family history, cystinuria, uric acid, RTA, hyperparathyroidism, milk-alkali sx, bone mets.

Investigation:

- IVP, U/S

Case 5.

40 YOM with severe abdominal pain, BP 90/60, P120. Assess and manage, heavy drinking the night before.

Case 6.

31 YOM presents in the ER curled up and tossing and in agonizing abdominal pain. Carry out the necessary examination and management. A nurse is helping you.

Key:

Talk to the patient for more information and give a running commentary as you examine.

Pay attention to patient situation: he is in shock BP90/60 and PR more than 100

Assessment:
- Do ABC, Vitals, BP sitting and supine
- Abdominal exam, search for rebound tenderness and signs of peritonitis, (pancreatitis or perforated bowel)

Management:
- Set IV, NS 1L runs in over 30 min
- Order blood tests including CBC, lytes, BUN Cr, Serum Ca^{2+} level, cross-match, amylase NG tube, Foley, oxygen, cardiac monitor
- Abdominal x-ray, U/S or CT
- General surgery consult
- Analgesia: IV meperidine 50 mg (after surgery consult)

Differential Diagnosis:
- Acute pancreatitis - Hx of binge drinking and Gastritis
- Perforated duodenum ulcer
- Acute cholecystitis

7. Thyroid mass

Case 1.

Middle aged female with thyroid mass. Obtain a history; what in the history indicates risks for malignancy?

Key: Diffuse enlargement versus nodules in thyroid, character of the nodule, associated symptoms.

History:
- *When did you notice the mass? Any changes overtime?*
- *Does the mass move when you swallow?*
- *Do you feel any discomfort in breathing, swallowing -compression symptom?*
- *Do you feel any pain?*
- *Do you have symptoms like heat intolerance, irritability, fine tremor, palpitation or diarrhea? -hyperthyroidism*
- *Do you have Symptoms like fatigue, cold intolerance, slowing of mental and physical activity or constipation? -- hypothyroidism*
- *Have you had irradiation to your head or neck for Acne?*
- *Do you have any family history of thyroid Ca?*
- *Rapid growth and failure to shrink on L-thyroxin*
- *Do you have any other lump(s) in your neck? Cervical lymphadenopathy*
- *Has your voice changed?*

History indicates malignancy:
- Firm, fixed nodule
- Voice change
- Rapid growth, no regression on L-thyroxin.
- Regional lymphadenopathy

Investigation:
- Fine needle aspiration
- Thyroid function test: TSH, free T4
- Thyroid scan
- U/S

8. Ankle Sprain

Case 1.
20 years old, sprained his ankle, assess and manage.

Key: Apply Ottawa ankle ruler to determine need for imaging.

Assessment:
- The position of ankle and foot at the time of the trauma for classification purpose: supination-adduction, supination-everstion (external rotation), pronation-abduction and pronation-eversion.
- Localization of tenderness, swelling, echymosis and deformity.
- Tests:Anterior drawer test, passive inversion
- Severity: 1st degree: stretching ligament fibers
  2nd degree: partial tear with pain and swelling
  3rd degree: Complete ligament separation

Diagnostic Studies:
- X-ray: PA, lateral, mortise.

Management:
RICE - Rest, Ice, Compression, Elevation

Control of swelling first
- Use elastic bandage, ice pack or ice water immerse 15-20 minutes, every 3-4 hrs x72 hrs. When awake, elevation of foot, analgesics

1st-2nd degree
- Repeat ice pack, after 72 hrs, change to hot soak
- Elastic bandage for 1-2 wks, neutral/slight everted position
- Partial weight bearing using a crutch until no pain
- Non-weight bearing exercise started 2-3 days include planter flexion, dorsal flexion, toe flexion, inversion, eversion

- After pain and swelling subside, weight bearing with sprain brace

3rd degree
- Surgical repair
- Cast immobilization 4-8 wks
- Refer to orthopedics

9. Abdominal Injury

Case 1.
Spleen trauma: Trauma code-what is your approach?

Case 2.
20 YOM in the ER, stabbed in the epigastria. BP 90/40, Manage.

Case 3.
A man is hit by a horse in the abdomen. He is in pain and tossing around. Do a physical exam. Write admitting orders regarding management.

Key:
Primary surgery – ABC, Brief History, Secondary Survey, definitive treatment

PE History resuscitation simultaneously

Management:
- ABC always first!
- Hi, I am Dr. X; I am here to help you, what happened for you? How do you feel?
  Doctor, I am in pain, I am stabbed! I am thirsty. Can I have some painkillers?
- Pay attention to, color (pale or cyanotic), sweating, respiratory distress (more than 36/min), agitation.
- Once happy with A+B, check vitals. If you couldn't sense the pulse in the hand, check the femoral pulse, but in this patient BP is more than 80 thus, you can sense the radial pulse. When ABC are OK, start to work on the patient, first with the establishment of IV line:
- Nurse please insert IV, size 16-gauge; the best solution is a crystalloid and rate of fluid depends on patients` clinical situation. If we need more than 2 litres for treatment of shock, we must consider blood transfusion.

Assessment:

- PE: Stabbing in the Epigastria requires you to pay special attention to the chest and abdomen cavities.   Check both sides of chest: for movement, breath sounds (pneumothorax, hemothorax), heart sounds (tamponad).
  Check Abdomen for local tenderness, rebound tenderness, assessment of wound, bowel sounds, and distention.
- Don't forget to do a DRE.
- Recheck ABC.
- Lab tests: Blood group, Cross match, Electrolytes, UA
- Don't forget to answer the patient:
  I am afraid you might have an internal injury, that involves bleeding or bowel perforation. You might need operations to fix the problem. So, see (be compassionate), I can't give you anything to drink but I'll do my best to keep you pain free.
- Check ABC, dropping BP, increase PR
- Can I have NG in, check GU, can I have Foley in?
- Surgery consults

10. Fall Trauma

Case 1.
A 30 YOM falls from a height of 10 metres. (1) tenderness in LUQ, (2) wound on left leg, (3) neck collar on, but asks for removal, (4) patient asks for analgesics. Manage.

Key:
Low blood pressure could be due to blood loss or spinal cord injury.

Intervention:
Primary survey and resuscitation:
a. Secure airway and C-spine
b. 100% Oxygen
c. IV line; if BP low, hydrate and prepare blood
Secondary Survey:
Mini Hx: From what height did he fall? How did the patient land? Was there any episode of loss of consciousness or amnesia? AMPLE.

Tertiary Survey: If admitted to hospital perform head to toe survey next day for missed injuries.

Assessment:
• Vitals
• Look for medical-alert tags, bracelets, necklace
• Head to toe survey.
• Looking for: tenderness over the spinous prosses, para spinal swelling, gap between spinous prosses (rupture of interspinous ligament)
• 3 X-rays: C-spine (AP, Lateral, Odontoid view), chest and, Pelvis X-rays
• Neurology: local signs, GCS

- Looking for: numbness or difficulty in limb movements, painless urinary retention, and priapism, urinary or fecal incontinence.
- Don't forget DRE.

Management:
Deal with problems in an orderly manner.
C-spine:
Clear C-spine if:
- No pain, no tenderness, No neurological signs and symptoms
- No significant distracting injury
- No head injury
- No intoxication
- X-ray: cleared

CT scan if there is problem in X-ray of neck or if there is neurological findings.
Spleen:
If vitals stable and no peritoneal sign, perform a CT scan of the abdomine and pelvis. FAST (focused abdominal sonography in trauma) examination may be used in unstable patients.
Wound:
Clean the wound and then suture; manage nerves, vessels and tendons damage, tetanus toxoid; antibiotics
Analgesics:
If vitals stable, LOC normal, clear C-spine, can have low dose of narcotic, but monitor closely.

11. Head Trauma

Case 1.
Head trauma, management

Key:
Never do lumbar puncture; always consider C-spine; don't blame coma on alcohol; low BP means injury elsewhere until proven otherwise, avoid overhydration (brain swelling).

Initial Management: ABCs
a. Airway with immobilization of C-spine suction, inline traction for nasal or endotracheal tube
- Talk to the pt, can talk – no tube, cannot talk – tube
- Contraindication for inserting nasal tubes in patients with major facial fractures. May require alternative strategies

b. 100% oxygen, head elevated (if T+L spines cleared)
- R/o: Airway obstruction, tension/open pneumothorax, massive hemothorax, cardiac tamponade, exanguinous active bleeding, flail chest – ATOM CEF

c. IV fluids, 2 large IV, NS or RL 2L bolus, maintaining BP (therefore central perfusion pressure) is important in head trauma.
- Differentiation of hypotensive shock (BP low, PR high) from neurogenic shock (BP low, PR low) is very important.
- Scan for obvious blood loss, NG, Foley
- Check vitals, ECG, blood work, ABG, glucose, toxicity screen, cross match blood, cardiac monitoring.

d. Spinal cord injury, early diagnose: weakness, numbness, and spinal pain, Quick assess GCS

e. Exposes the patient (all clothes off).

Initial Assessment:
Mini history:
- From witness, ambulance attendants, family-circumstances, mechanism of injury, seat belt on? Where was he found, hit

windshield, period of LOC loss, post traumatic amnesia, loss of sensation/function, AMPLE

Predisposing factors: any meds-pill box in car, drug hx, psychiatric hx, seizure, poor vision, head or neck pain, laceration, LOC, change in breath pattern, double or blurred vision, N/V, urinary or fecal incontinence, ability to move all extremities

Head to toe survey:

- Identify major injuries
- Tubes and fingers in every orifice
- Med-Alert tags, splint fractures
- Look for specific toxidromes
- 5N's: Noggin (Racoon eyes, Battle's sign), Neck (c-spine) ENT, Needle (tracks for drug abuse), Neurological
- Neck– open collar if calm, check: C-spine, trachea, JVP

Neurology Exam:

- LOC – Glasgow coma scale
- Head/neck: Laceration, bruises, basal skull fracture (hematoma around Eyes or behind ears), facial fracture foreign body
- To identify CSF: double ring sign on a blotting paper: inside ring-blood, outside ring CSF
- Signs of increased ICP: Hiccup, yawn, Cushing's reflex (BP up, PR low), breath pattern, pupil size and reactivity, extra ocular movement, nystagmus, fundoscopy.
- Brain stem:
  Cranial nerve palsy, breath pattern, doll's eye phenomenon
- Spine:
  Deformity, tenderness
- Motor:
  Can he move his fingers/toes, muscle tone, power, sensitivity-if unconscious, test response to pain/stimulation, reflex-corneal, abdomen, and sphincter tone, squeeze nail bed, check reflex of Achilles tendon.

Other significant trauma:

Must rule out abdominal and perineal trauma, flail chest, pneumothorax/hemothorax, cardiac tamponade, active bleeding-shock

Investigation:

- Cervical, Thoracic and, Lumbar spine X-ray. AP lateral, odontoid views for C-spine must see C1-T1. Alignment, Bone, cartilage and Soft Tissue
- CT head and upper C-spine
- CXR, ABG, CBC, drug screen
- Neurosurgery consult

Late Management:

Minor head injury: observe 24-48 hrs, wake up every hr, no sedatives or painkillers

Severe head injury:

1. Make sure ABCs and monitor neurological sign
2. Elevated ICP: manitol 1g/kg IV then OR, elevation of head and, hyperventilation
3. Surgery: removal of hematoma (Neurosurgery)

Spinal Injury:

1. Reduce dislocation by traction or surgery, stabilize.
2. Emergent surgical decompression and/or fusion may be required.

Continue Care:

Continue evaluation and therapy, specific consultations like surgery, disposition-home, and admission to ICU

12. Suture Laceration

Case 1.
Suture scalp and skin laceration.

General Considerations:
- Always consider every structure deep to laceration served until proved otherwise.
- Think about anatomy, never test function against resistance.
- Examine tendon and neurovascular status distal to laceration.
- X-ray for foreign body if necessary.
- Clean and explore under local anesthetic

Management:
- Wash hands, wear gloves.
- Apply local anesthesia, LET, no epinephrine in certain areas, (Fingers, Ears and, Nose)
- Irrigate the wound copiously with NS.
- Give pain killer, stop bleeding with direct pressure over the wound. NEVER try to control bleeding with clamping because there is always possibility of damage to nerves. If you have any problem, call a plastic or general surgeon.
- Prepare the field with betadine; drape the wound with sterile cloth.
- Debride dead tissue/foreign body (the best way for debridment is using a sharp device like surgical Mets 'scissors' or a scalpel)
- Suture deep tissue with absorbable material: Catgut, Dexon, Vycril (for subcutaneous)
- Skin: Nylon: face 6-0, scalp 3-4 0, trunk or extremity, 4-5 0, Joint surface 4-5 0, 2-3 mm apart, 2-3 mm edge.
- Small vessels-plain catgut; large vessels-chromic catgut. Plain catgut is absorbed more quickly than chromic catgut.
- Splinting, internal or external fixation for fractures, anastmosis of important blood vessels and nerve.

Post-suture:

a. Dress wound, remove dressing after 24 hrs, may shower in 1-2 days

b. Tetanus Prophylaxis:

Immunization History	non-Tetanus Prone wounds		Tetanus prone*	
	Td	TIG	Td	TIG
Uncertain or<3 doses.........	Yes	No	Yes	Yes
3 or more, none for>10 years	Yes	No	Yes	No
3 or more, >5 but <10 years	No	No	Yes	No
3 or more, <4 years ago	No	No	No	No

*wounds >6 hours old, >1cm deep, puncture wounds, avulsions, wounds resulting from missiles, crush wounds, burns, frost bite, wounds contaminated with dirt, soil or saliva.

c. Antibiotics, Local polysporine ointment PRN if only skin
• Systemic antibiotics if bone, tendon, or joint space penetrated

d. Check circulation, nerve-sensation/movement

e. Remove suture: joint 14-21 POD (depends on place of joint. For example knee joints or MCP joints), face 3-5 POD, other 7 POD, oral mucosa 10-14, scalp 5-7 POD

Case 2.

20 YOM has lacerated his right forearm on a broken beer bottle. Obtain a history, do a physical exam and manage.

History:

• *When, Where and How (mechanism) – position, direction, power?*
• *Hand dominance, occupation, hobbies?*
• *Visible arterial spurting at the time of injury?*
• *Previous hand trauma/surgery?*
• *Tetanus, Meds, allergy?*
• *Any other injury? Dizziness? Headache? hemodynamically stable?*

Physical Exam:

Inspect: Deformity, depth and range of laceration, active bleeding, and color. Pale/blue, swelling, bruising, perfusion

Palpate: Pulse, temperature, and sensation

ROM: Be careful DON'T test function against resistance.

Nerve: Sensory loss

Motor-extrinsic muscles, intrinsic muscles, superficial, and profound

Sympathetic (sweating)

Vessel: Capillary refill, Allen test, color, turgor, temperature

Tendon: Don't test against resistance

Management:

Nerve: Clean cut, <24 hr, no concurrent major injury, repair, epineural with minimum tension, F/U 3w and 6wks

Physiotherapy to prevent joint contracture

Vessel: Control bleeding with direct pressure and hand elevation

Avoid probing, clamping or tying off to avoid nerve injury

<6 hr, repair

Dressing, immobilize, and splint with fingertips visible

Monitor: color, turgor, capillary refill and temperature

Tendon: Most require primary repair, never test against resistance, never immobilize for more than 3 weeks to avoid stiffness

Case 3.

A man fell on a nail. He is a construction worker. He has injured his forearm. Neurovascular bundles are normal. Wound is cleaned and ready for you.

Management:

- First try to irrigate the wound with N\S. After meticulous irrigation, start to prepare and drape the wound to begin suturing.
- Use sterile suture #5, toothed forceps, gloves and local anesthesia 1% xylocaine.

The examiner will ask you:

Q: What will you do after bandaging?

- Wide spectrum antibiotics.
- Check his tetanus status.
- F/U every other day with dressing.
- check neurovascular status before/after suture.

Q: When are you going to remove the stitches?
- 1 wk to 10 days.

Case 4.

A young man who had just finished his exam went out celebrating and got drunk. He injured his wrist with a bottle. Do a physical exam.

Key:

Don't examine against resistance.
Ask about his occupation and if he is left or right handed.

Diagnosis:

Median nerve injury

Q: What are the 4 structures that severed?
A: Superficial: Flexor capri ulnaris, flexor capri radialis, palmaris longus;
Deep: Flexor digitorium superficialis, flexor digitorium profundus Adductor pollicis longus,
Nerve: median nerve, ulnar nerve
Vessels: radial artery, ulnar artery

Q: Why is the thumb weak?
A: Median nerve
- Adductor polices brevis opposition

13. Motor Vehicle Accident

Case 1.
22 YOM was driving a motorcycle when a car hit him. He was thrown 20 metres. He is brought into the ER in a coma and with a cervical collar. Assess the patient.

Key:
ABCs, mini history, secondary survey see case 10 and 11.
Specific issues for MVA addressed here.

Motor vehicle collisions:
- Weight and size of vehicle
- Speed of vehicle.
- Site of anatomic impact.
- Use of helmet.
- Type of crash and associated serious injuries:
  a. Lateral (T-bone): head, cervical spine, thoracic and abdominal injuries.
  b. Front end: head, cervical spine, thoracic, abdominal, pelvic and lower extremities.
  c. Rear end: over extension of cervical spine, (whiplash injury to neck).
  d. Ejection of patient from vehicle or entrapment of patient under vehicle.
- Location of patient in vehicle.
- Death of any other passenger, traveling with that car.
- Degree of damage to vehicle especially if intrusion into passenger compartment.
- Seat belt, airbags?
  Lap belt: look for lower spine and abdominal injury.
  Shoulder belt: look for major vessel injury.
- Any loss of consciousness, for how long? Amnesia?
- Head injury, vomiting, headache? Seizure?
- Use of alcohol, illicit drugs?

Q: Is this x-ray view enough?

Q: Describe the abnormalities seen.

Q: There is serosanguinous clear nasal discharge. What is the significance of this discharge?

• Fracture of the base of the skull

Q: What other investigations will you do on this serosanguinous fluid?

• Avoid nasal and ear packing; consider C+S. Consider use of prophylactic antibiotic in case of otorhea (base skull fracture)

14. Burn

Case 1.
Burn victim. Manage.

Key:
Avoid nasal and ear packing, consider C+S.
* same principle as other trauma with some exceptions e.g., Tetanus, fluid resuscitation, inhalation injury

Management:
a. Ensure burning process has stopped, remove synthetic fabrics, clothes in hot water
b. Airway and Breathing ? watch for upper airway edema
Factors suggesting inhalation injury:
* Confinement in a burning building
* Explosion
* Lost consciousness
* Carbon deposits around nose or mouth, throat.
* Inflammatory changes in oropharynx
* Change in voice
* Carbon in sputum
* Curled facial hair
c. Circulation: 2 large bore IV in upper extremity, go through burned skin if have to, >20% burn need IV support.
4 cc/kg/surface area of 2nd to 3rd degree burn.
d. Complete primary survey, start secondary survey
* Look for other injury, remove jewelery to prevent circulatory compromise, escharotomy or faciotomy
* Pain control
* Systemic antibiotics
* Wound care, cover with sterile dressing, topical silver sulfadiazine, polysporine for face.

15. Testicular Pain

Case.

17 YOM complains of testicular pain, take a focused history.

Key:

DDx include trauma, Infection (mumps, orcheitis), epididymitis, testicular torsion, torsion of epididymal cyst

- *Was the pain preceded by trauma?*
- *How rapidly did the pain develop?*
- *Was the pain preceded by fever or swelling of the salivary glands (mumps)?*
- *Was it associated with burning on micturition or a urethral discharge?*

Acronyms

AA	amino acid
AAA	abdominal aorta aneurysm
Ab	antibody
ABC	airways, breathing, circulation
ABG	arterial blood gas
ABI	ankle-brachial index
AC	acromioclavicular joint
ACE	angiotensin converting enzyme
ACEI	angiotensin converting enzyme inhibitor
ACLS	advanced cardiac life support
A/E	aspiration/exhalation
Ag	antigen
AMPLE	allergies, medications, past medical history, last menstrual period, events
ANA	anti-nuclear antibody
AS	ankylosing spondylitis
ASA	acetylsalicylic acid or aspirin
ASO	anti-streptolysin O
AVM	arterial venous malformation
BCP	birth control pills
BM	bowel movement
BP	blood pressure
BPH	benign prostate hypertrophy
BPP	biophysical profile
BPPV	benign paroxysmal positional vertigo
BUN	blood urea nitrogen
Ca	cancer, carcinoma
Ca^{2+}	calcium
CAD	coronary artery disease
cAMP	cyclic adenosine monophosphate
CBC	complete blood count
C/D	constipation/diarrhea
CHF	congestive heart failure
CK-MB	creatinine kinase-MB

CNS	central nervous system
C/O	complains of
Cr	creatinine
C+S	culture and sensitivity
CSA	child support agency
CT	computer tomography
CTS	carpal tunnel syndrome
CVA	costovertebrae angle
CVD	cardiovascular disease
CVS	chorionic villi sampling
CXR	chest x-ray
D/C	discontinue
D+C	dilation and curettage
DDx	differential diagnosis
DKA	diabetic ketoacidosis
DM	diabetes mellitus
DRE	digital rectal exam
DPTP	diphtheria, acellular pertussis, tetanus, inactivated polio vaccine
DUB	dysfunctional uterine bleeding
DTR	deep tendon reflex
DVT	deep venous thrombosis
EDD	expected date of delivery
ENG	electronystagmography
ER	emergency room, estrogen receptor
ESR	erythrocyte sedimentation rate
ETOH	ethanol, alcohol
FAST	focused abdominal sonography in trauma
FDP	fibrinogen degradation product
F-E	flexion-extension
FFA	free fatty acid
FHR	fetal heart rate
FHx	family history
FNA	fine needle aspiration
FSH	follicular stimulating hormone
FTT	failure to thrive
GBS	group B streptococcus

GC	gonococcus
GCS	glagow coma scale
GERD	gastroesophageal reflux disease
GH	glenohumeral joint
GI	gastrointestinal tract
GMC	general medical condition
GP	general practitioner
G&P	gravidity and parity
GTPAL	gravidity, term infants, parity, abortion, living children
GU	genitourinary
HB	hemoglobin
HEENT	head, eyes, ears, nose and throat
HiB	hemophillius influenza type B conjugate vaccine
HPF	high power field
HPV	human papilloma virus
HRT	hormone replacement therapy
HTN	hypertension
HUS	hemolytic uremic syndrome
HVS	hysterovaginal scope
IBD	inflammatory bowel disease
ICP	introcranial pressure
IDDM	insulin-dependent diabetes mellitus
I-E	internal-external rotation
IHD	ischemic heart disease
INH	isoniazid
INR	international normalized ratio
IPPA	inspection, palpation, percussion, ausculation
ITP	idiopathic thrombocytopenic purpura
IUD	intrauterine device
IUGR	intrauterine growth retardation
IVP	intravenous pyelogram
JVP	jugular vein pressure
KFTs	kidney function tests
KUB	kidney ureter bladder
LET	lidocaine, epinephrine, tetracaine
LF	liver failure
LFT	liver function test

LH	luteinizing hormone
LLQ	left lower quadrant
LMN	lower motor neuron
LMP	last menstrual period
LN	lymph node
LOC	level of consciousness
LRT	lower respiratory tract
L/S	lumbar/sacral
LUQ	left upper quadrant
LVF	left ventricular failure
MCV	mean corpuscular volume
MEN	multiple endocrine neoplasia
MMR	measles, mumps, rubella
MMSE	minimum mental status exam
MSE	mental status exam
MSK	musculoskeletal
MSS	maternal serum screen
MSU	midstream urine (sample)
MVA	motor vehicle accident
NAVEL	nerve, artery, vein, empty space, lymph node
NCV	nerve conduction velocity
NG	nasogastric tube
NPO	nil per os
NS	normal saline
NSAID	nonsteroidal anti-inflammatory drugs
NST	non-stress test
N/V	nausea and vomiting
OA	osteoarthritis
OGCT	oral glucose challenge test
OLDCARS	onset, location, duration, cause, associated symptoms, radiation, severity.
O + P	ova and parasites
OPQRST	onset, precipitating/alleviating factors, quality, radiation, site, timing
OPV	oral polio vaccine
OR	operating room
PAP	Prostate acid phosphatase

PCP	pnemacystitis carinii pneumonia
PE	physical examination, pulmonary embolism
PFT	pulmonary function test
PID	pelvic inflammatory disease
PMHx	past medical history
PND	paroxysmal nocturnal dyspnea
POD	post operative day
PR	pulse rate
PRH	prolactin hormone
PRN	as needed
PSA	prostate specific antigen
PTCA	percutaneous transluminal coronary angioplasty
PTH	parathyroid hormone
PLP	PTH-like protein
PT	prothrombin time
PTT	partial thromboplastin time
PUD	peptic ulcer disease
PV	per vaginal
RA	rheumatoid arthritis
RBC	red blood cells
RF	renal failure
RLQ	right lower quardrant
R/O	rule out
ROM	range of motion
RR	respiratory rate
RTA	renal tubular acidosis
SC	sternoclavicular joint
S/C	subcutaneous injection
Scr	serum creatinine
SEADS	swelling, erythema, atrophy, deformity, skin changes
SEM	systolic ejection murmur
SHx	social history
SI	sacroiliac joint
SLE	systemic lupus erythematosus
ST	scapulothoracic joint
STD	sexual transmitted disease
SOB	shortness of breath

SPEP	serum protein electrophoresis
Sx	symptoms
TB	tuberculosis
TdP	tetanus, diphteria toxoid, and polio
THR	total hip replacement
TIA	transient ischemia attack
TIG	tetanus immune globulin
TMJ	temporomandibular joint
TRUS	transrectal ultrasound
TSH	thyroid stimulating hormone
TSS	toxic shock syndrome
Tx	treatment
UA	urine analysis
UMN	upper motor neuron
UPEP	urine protein electrophoresis
URTI	upper respiratory tract infection
U/S	ultrasound
UTI	urinary tract infection
VATS	video-assisted thoracoscopy
VBI	vertebrobasilar insufficiency
VDRL	veneral disease research laboratory
YO	year old